Infection Control

and

OSHA Essentials

Infection Control

and

OSHA Essentials

Fifth Edition

BARBARA S. RUSSELL, RN, MPH, CIC, ACRN
DIRECTOR, INFECTION CONTROL SERVICES
BAPTIST HOSPITAL
MIAMI, FLORIDA

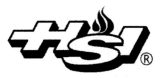

Health Studies Institute, Inc.

iUniverse, Inc.
New York   Bloomington

Infection Control and OSHA Essentials

The information, ideas, and suggestions in this book are not intended as a substitute for professional medical advice. Before following any suggestions contained in this book, you should consult your personal physician. Neither the author nor the publisher shall be liable or responsible for any loss or damage allegedly arising as a consequence of your use or application of any information or suggestions in this book.

iUniverse books may be ordered through booksellers or by contacting:

iUniverse
1663 Liberty Drive
Bloomington, IN 47403
www.iuniverse.com
1-800-Authors (1-800-288-4677)

Because of the dynamic nature of the Internet, any Web addresses or links contained in this book may have changed since publication and may no longer be valid. The views expressed in this work are solely those of the author and do not necessarily reflect the views of the publisher, and the publisher hereby disclaims any responsibility for them.

ISBN: 978-1-4401-2569-0 (sc)
ISBN: 978-1-4401-2568-3 (ebk)

Printed in the United States of America

iUniverse rev. date: 5/19/2009

Barbara S. Russell, RN, MPH, CIC, ACRN, is Director of Infection Control Services at Baptist Hospital of Miami, Florida, and the Co-Chair of Baptist Health South Florida's System Emergency Operations Council. She has specialized in infection control for over 30 years and is Infection Control Certified. She is the 2002 recipient of the City of Miami Chamber of Commerce Health Professional Hero of the Year Award and the Carol DeMille Achievement Award, presented by the Association for Professionals in Infection Control and Epidemiology (APIC), for her outstanding contributions to infection control and patient care.

Barbara was the 1997 recipient of the Association of Nurses in AIDS Care (ANAC) National Leadership Award. In 1994, she was President of the National APIC, and, in 1999, President of the National Federation of Specialty Nursing Organizations (NFSNO). She has also served as Chair of both the Florida Nurses Association and the American Nurses Association HIV Task Forces. In 1988, she was one of 14 U.S. nurses to receive a Certificate of Commendation from the Assistant Secretary of Health and Human Services for her work on AIDS.

Ms. Russell has testified before the Occupational Safety and Health Administration (OSHA), Centers for Disease Control and Prevention (CDC), State of Florida legislators, and three U.S. Congressional subcommittees on behalf of health care worker safety. She actively promotes education and safer work environments, and has written numerous articles for professional newsletters and journals.

Dental Consultant: Wendy S. Hupp, DMD, is an Assistant Professor and the Director of Oral Medicine, Department of Diagnostic Sciences, College of Dental Medicine, Nova Southeastern University, Fort Lauderdale, Florida. Dr. Hupp is a Diplomate of the American Board of Oral Medicine.

Dr. Hupp earned her DMD at the University of Pennsylvania School of Dental Medicine. Her numerous presentations on clinical oral diagnosis, medicine, and pathology include those on oral cancer and tobacco cessation, aphthous ulcers, dental pharmacology, viral hepatitis, human immunodeficiency virus, seizure disorders, and women's health.

Cover design: Rob Johnson.

Contents

Introduction **13**

    Current Challenges... 13

        Emerging and Re-emerging Infections.................................. 13

        Drug-Resistant Pathogens.. 14

    CDC Guidelines.. 14

        General Infection Control.. 14

        Preexposure and Postexposure Prophylaxis....................... 15

    Health Care Workers' Responsibilities 16

        Understanding the Cycle of Infection 16

        Preventing Infection in the Workplace................................ 17

        Learning and Sharing Information 18

Chapter 1   The Infection Process **21**

    Cycle of Infection 21

        Reservoirs.. 22

        Exit Vehicles.. 22

        Transmission Modes 22

        Entry Portals... 25

        Susceptible Hosts.. 25

    Interrupting the Infection Process.. 26

        Standard Precautions 27

        Transmission-Based Precautions 28

Chapter 2   Overview of Bacteria and Protozoans..............................33

Bacillus anthracis 34

Bordetella pertussis 35

Chlamydia pneumoniae 36

Clostridium botulinum 36

Clostridium difficile 37

Corynebacterium diphtheriae 38

Cryptosporidium parvum 39

Escherichia coli Serotype O157:H7 39

Giardia lamblia 40

Legionella pneumophila 41

Mycobacterium tuberculosis 41

Mycoplasma pneumoniae 45

Neisseria meningitidis (Meningococcus)...................... 45

Salmonella enterica 46

Shigella sonnei 47

Staphylococcus aureus 48

Streptococcus pneumoniae (Pneumococcus)................. 49

Streptococcus pyogenes 49

Toxoplasma gondii 51

Vancomycin-Resistant Enterococcus (VRE) 51

Chapter 3   Overview of Viruses 55

Adenoviruses.. 55

Cytomegalovirus 56

Hepatitis A Virus 57

Hepatitis B Virus.. 58

Hepatitis C Virus.. 61

Other Hepatitis Viruses 62

Herpes Simplex Viruses.. 62

Human Immunodeficiency Virus (HIV).......................... 63

Influenza Viruses 66

Mumps Virus.. 67

Norovirus... 68

Polioviruses.. 68

Respiratory Syncytial Virus.. 69

Rubella Virus 70

Rubeola Virus 71

Varicella Zoster Virus 72

Variola Virus 73

Chapter 4   Occupational Exposure Responses 77

Postexposure Responses 77

OSHA Requirements 79

Ethical Obligations 79

Chapter 5   At-Work Personal Infection Control 81

Handwashing and Hand Antisepsis 81

Hand-Cleansing Methods and Agents 83

Routine Handwashing 83

Hand Antisepsis 84

Surgical Hand Scrub 84

Hand-Cleansing Products 84

Personal Protective Equipment 86

Protective Gloves 86

OSHA-Required Inhalation and Eye Protection 92

Types of Inhalation Protection 92

Types of Eye protection 95

Special Dentistry Barriers 96

Protective Clothing 96

Other Personal Infection Control 98

Chapter 6   Sterilizing Instruments 99

Susceptibility of Microbes 99

Instrument Classifications 100

Sterilants and Their Uses 100

Dry Heat 101

Ethylene Oxide 104

Glutaraldehydes 104

Hydrogen Peroxide 104

Peracetic Acid 104

Steam 105

Unsaturated Chemical Vapor 106

Sterilization Steps 106

Presoaking Instruments (Step 1) 106

Precleaning Instruments (Step 2) 107

Packaging Instruments (Step 3) 109

Loading Sterilizers (Step 4) 109

Monitoring Sterilization (Step 5) 110

Handling and Storing Sterilized Instruments (Step 6) 113

Sterilizer Cleaning 114

Chain of Events in Clinical Settings 114

Chapter 7 Disinfection **117**

High-Level Disinfection 117

Intermediate- and Low-Level Disinfection................................. 118

Protective Coverings.. 121

Special Disinfecting Procedures.. 122

Endoscope Disinfection 123

Dental Unit Water Line Disinfection.................................... 124

Dental Material Disinfection 125

Dental Radiographic Equipment.. 126

Chapter 8 Hazard Controls **128**

Sharps: Handle with Care! 128

Tips on Sharps in General.. 129

Tips on Use and Disposal of Needles.................................... 131

Regulated Waste 133

Containers 134

Warning and Identification Labels.. 134

Disposal of Regulated Waste.. 135

Liquid Waste 136

Hazardous Chemicals 136

Hazard Reporting 138

Chapter 9 Planning and Training **140**

Exposure Control Plan 140

Infection Control Manager 140

Employee Medical Evaluations 142

Employee Training 142

Bloodborne Pathogens.. 142

All Contagious Diseases 143

Hazardous Chemicals..143
Training Methods 145
Required Documents 145

Chapter 10 Record Keeping **147**
Employee Medical Records 147
OSHA Logs 147
Logs 300 and 301..148
Sharps Injury Log 148
Training Records...149

Definitions **151**

Appendix A   Information Sources...**161**

Appendix B   Preexposure Vaccination Checklist for U.S. Residents **163**

Appendix C   Infection Control Checklist: Outpatient Clinical Practices.....**169**

Appendix D   Disease Spread in Dental Offices..**171**

Index..**174**

Reference List for Further Study..**184**

Algorithms

Algorithm 1. Standard and Transmission-Based Precautions 29
Algorithm 2. Allergic Reactions to Natural Rubber Latex................................91
Algorithm 3. Masks and N95 or HEPA Personal Respirators 95

Figures

Fig. 1. Cycle of Infection..23
Fig. 2. Hazardous Bioaerosols..31
Fig. 3. Eyewash Station Capped 78
Fig. 4. Eyewash Station Operating..78
Fig. 5. N95 Particulate Respirator and Surgical Mask................................93
Fig. 6. Vented HEPA Respirator 93
Fig. 7. Steam Autoclave 105
Fig. 8. Ultrasonic Cleaner 107
Fig. 9. Biological Monitoring..111

Fig. 10. Disposable Plastic Surface Barriers..122
Fig. 11. Operating Light with Plastic Cover..123
Fig. 12. Don't Do This!...130
Fig. 13. The Scoop Technique...132
Fig. 14. Needle Recapping Stand...132
Fig. 15. Sharps Container 134

Tables

Table 1. Tuberculosis Infection Control Checklist.............................. 43
Table 2. Hepatitis B Vaccine and OSHA Compliance 59
Table 3. Hepatitis B Virus Postexposure Prophylaxis (PEP) Guidelines.......... 60
Table 5. Bloodborne Pathogen Exposures and OSHA Compliance 80
Table 6. Handwashing and OSHA Compliance...................................... 82
Table 7. Hand Antisepsis and Surgical Hand Scrub Steps 85
Table 8. Antimicrobial Agents in Hand-Cleansing Products................... 87
Table 9. Personal Protective Equipment and OSHA Compliance.................. 88
Table 10. Gloves and OSHA Compliance 89
Table 11. Gloves Used in Health Care Settings..................................... 90
Table 12. Masks and Eye Protection—OSHA Compliance...................... 92
Table 13. Protective Clothing, Laundry, and OSHA Compliance 97
Table 14. Critical- and Semicritical-Class Instruments or Devices............... 101
Table 15. Sterilants and Characteristics of Their Use 102
Table 16. Presoaking Procedures 107
Table 17. Precleaning Procedures 108
Table 18. Instrument Packaging Procedures 109
Table 19. Sodium Hypochlorite... 118
Table 20. Iodophors and Phenolics.. 119
Table 21. Housekeeping and OSHA Compliance 120
Table 22. Sharps and OSHA Compliance 129
Table 23. Regulated Waste and OSHA Compliance 133
Table 24. Biohazard Warning Labels and OSHA Compliance..................... 135
Table 25. Exposure Control Plan and OSHA Compliance 141
Table 26. Employee Training and OSHA Compliance 144
Table 27. Confidential Employee Medical Records & OSHA Compliance... 148

Introduction

Although many of the approximately 9 million health care workers in the United States are employed in hospitals, more and more are serving in nursing homes, outpatient and emergency care clinics, and patients' homes. <u>Any</u> person providing health care can acquire infections from, or transmit infections to, patients, coworkers, household members, and/or other community contacts. Health care providers can also spread infections from patient to patient.

To protect themselves, their patients, and others from infection, health care workers should consistently use Occupational Safety and Health Administration (OSHA)-required and Centers for Disease Control and Prevention (CDC)-recommended infection control strategies. By doing so, they can interrupt the infection process *(see Chapter 1, Interrupting the Infection Process).*

Current Challenges

Emerging and Re-emerging Infections

Infections are caused by pathogens (disease-producing microbes) that enter human bodies via various routes *(see Chapter 1, Fig. 1).* Health care workers' efforts to prevent infections are often hindered by the pace at which they must work and the numbers and kinds of pathogens they encounter. During recent decades, health care workers have been confronted with: (1) many newly recognized pathogens (e.g., hepatitis C and human immunodeficiency viruses), and (2) many re-emerging infections (e.g., those caused by *Escherichia coli* serotype O157:H7, *Bordetella pertussis,* group A streptococcus, and *Salmonella enterica).* This book provides infection control overviews for these infections, as well as many others, including those caused by *Bacillus anthracis* (a significant challenge to health care workers since 2001) and *Clostridium botulinum* and variola virus (which have potential for bioterrorist use).

Drug-Resistant Pathogens

The resistance of many pathogens to antimicrobials has created serious therapeutic dilemmas worldwide. Penicillin-resistant *Streptococcus pneumoniae* poses problems in treating pneumonia and meningitis caused by this bacterium. Vancomycin-resistant enterococci (especially *Enterococcus faecalis)* also pose problems, and *Staphylococcus aureus,* already resistant to methicillin, has the potential to become vancomycin-resistant. The resistance of *Mycobacterium tuberculosis* to drugs traditionally used to treat tuberculosis makes multidrug regimens necessary for infected patients. Some strains of influenza virus type A are now resistant to amantadine and rimantadine. To prevent development of drug-resistant pathogens, clinicians must prescribe antimicrobials appropriately and urge patients to complete their drug regimens.

CDC Guidelines

Despite these many challenges, progress is being made in the fight against infectious diseases. The CDC constantly raises its infection control standards; new guidelines can be downloaded from the www.cdc.gov/ncidod website. Some CDC guidelines are listed below *(see this book's Reference List for complete information).* Readers should obtain all relevant documents and keep abreast of future updates.

General Infection Control

1. *Guideline for Infection Control in Healthcare Personnel.*[1] This guideline applies to all paid and unpaid persons working in health

care settings who have the potential for exposure to infectious materials, including body substances, contaminated medical supplies and equipment, contaminated environmental surfaces, and/or contaminated air. These workers include, but are not limited to, dental, mortuary, laboratory, and emergency medical service personnel, nurses and nursing assistants, physicians, technicians, students and trainees, contractual staff not directly employed by health care facilities, and clerical, dietary, housekeeping, maintenance, and volunteer personnel of health care facilities (if they might be exposed to infectious agents).

2. *Guideline for Isolation Precautions in Hospitals.* This guideline describes use of Standard and Transmission-Based Precautions.[2] The same precautions can be applied in outpatient facilities (e.g., protecting dental professionals from patients with herpes lesions, or sequestering coughing patients who might transmit airborne diseases).

3. *Guidelines for Preventing Transmission of* Mycobacterium tuberculosis *in Health-Care Facilities.*[3]

4. *Guidelines for the Prevention of Surgical Site Infection, 1999.*[4]

5. *Guidelines for Prevention of Intravascular Catheter-Related Infections, 2002.*[5]

6. *Recommendations for Preventing Transmission of Infections Among Chronic Hemodialysis Patients.*[6]

7. *Guideline for Hand Hygiene in Health-Care Settings, 2002.*[7]

8. *Management of Multidrug-Resistant Organisms in Healthcare Settings, 2006.*[8]

9. *Guidelines for Infection Control in Dental Health Care Settings— 2003.*[9]

Preexposure and Postexposure Prophylaxis

1. *Updated U.S. Public Health Service Guidelines for the Management of Occupational Exposures to HBV, HCV, and HIV and Recommendations for Postexposure Prophylaxis.*[10]

2. *Immunization of Health-Care Workers,*[11] and *Recommended Immunization Schedules for Persons Aged 0–18 Years–United States, 2007.*[12]

3. *Recommendations for the Use of Antiretroviral Drugs in Pregnant HIV-Infected Women for Maternal Health and Interventions to Reduce Perinatal HIV-1 Transmission in the United States.*[13]

4. *Prevention of Pneumococcal Disease,*[14] and *Preventing Pneumococcal Disease Among Infants and Young Children.*[15]

5. *Guidelines for Prevention of Nosocomial Pneumonia.*[16]

6. *Prevention and Control of Influenza.*[17]

7. *Prevention and Control of Meningococcal Disease,* and *Meningococcal Disease and College Students.*[18]

8. *Poliomyelitis Prevention in the United States.*[19]

9. *Control and Prevention of Rubella.*[20]

10. *Prevention of Varicella.*[21]

Health care workers should also be familiar with the American Heart Association's current guidelines for prevention of bacterial endocarditis (available at www.americanheart.org).

Health Care Workers' Responsibilities

Health care workers are obligated to eliminate or at least reduce pathogen transmission in their clinical practices, hospitals, and other health care settings and research laboratories. This book reviews the methods necessary to achieve this goal.

Understanding the Cycle of Infection

Health care workers should understand the cycle of infection *(see Chapter 1, Fig. 1)* and how use of appropriate precautions in the workplace can interrupt this cycle. Basic knowledge about the bacteria, protozoans, and viruses encountered in health care settings is vital to fighting infection. Chapters 2 and 3 describe the infectious substances involved in the transmission of more than 30 of these pathogens, as well as the contagion periods.

Workers should also know that fungi (e.g., *Aspergillus fumigatus, Candida albicans, Coccidioides immitis, Cryptococcus neoformans,* and *Histoplasma capsulatum*) frequently cause infections in immuno<u>compromised</u> patients. Immuno<u>competent</u> health care workers are not usually at risk of acquiring such infections, but they should use Standard Precautions *(described in Chapter 1)* when caring for patients with fungal infections. Other precautions include keeping health care facilities dust- and mildew-free and properly disinfected. For example, fungi can be transmitted in air flowing through ventilation systems, nonsterile water used in medical equipment, and dust emanating from surfaces disturbed during repair or construction work. The CDC 2003 guidelines for environmental infection control in health care facilities addresses these problems.[22]

Preventing Infection in the Workplace

Chapters 2 and 3 also describe, for more than 30 kinds of pathogens, the appropriate respiratory (Airborne or Droplet) and/or isolation (Standard and Contact) precautions; factors that increase infection risks; available vaccines and postexposure treatments; case reporting; and work restrictions. Chapter 4 focuses on responses to occupational exposures to pathogens, including immediate first aid and, for bloodborne pathogen exposures, OSHA-required confidential medical evaluations.

Chapters 5 through 8 describe OSHA-required and CDC-recommended infection control procedures to be used in health care facilities. Some states and territories administer their own occupational safety and health programs *(see Appendix A),* which must meet or exceed the OSHA requirements dealing with occupational exposure to bloodborne pathogens.[23] Health care workers should know the provisions of their state programs, as well as specific state regulations, including those of occupational licensing boards, health departments, and environmental agencies. Infection control procedures are also affected by many local (county or city) regulations.

The OSHA requirements discussed in this book apply to all health care workers. However, those working in hepatitis B and human immunodeficiency virus research facilities should consult Section 1910.1030(e) of OSHA's "Occupational Exposure to Bloodborne Pathogens; Final Rule" for <u>further</u> requirements.[23] These include special training for laboratory employees, as well as use of certified biological safety cabinets and centrifuges that can be locked before their operation and have safety cups and sealed rotors.

This text concludes with descriptions of OSHA-required exposure control plans, new employee medical evaluations, employee training, and record keeping *(see Chapters 9 and 10).*

Learning and Sharing Information

After completing this course, health care workers should:

1. Continue to update their knowledge by checking frequently with their Infection Control Managers, and by consulting the CDC website (www.cdc.gov) and medical journals.

2. Routinely tell their patients how to avoid and/or halt the spread of infectious diseases.

3. Educate new caregivers on the use of appropriate respiratory (Airborne or Droplet) and/or isolation (Standard and Contact) precautions (e.g., hospital staff should do this before transferring infected patients to nursing homes or releasing them to go home). The new caregivers should know how the patients' infections can be transmitted and what precautions will protect other patients, health care workers, and/or family members from acquiring those infections.

4. Have a written infection control plan in place to minimize the risk of disease transmission among health care workers and their patients.

5. Dental offices should establish referral arrangements with qualified health care professionals to ensure prompt and appropriate provision of preventive services, occupationally related medical services, and postexposure management with medical follow-up.

Notes:

1. For infection control information on communicable diseases not discussed in this book, readers should call their local health departments, consult books such as *Control of Communicable Diseases Manual*,[24] or refer to the www.cdc.gov website where, for example, information on sexually transmitted diseases can be

found in *Morbidity and Mortality Weekly Report,* 11(RR-55) dated August 4, 2006.

2. Further information on pathogens with potential for bioterrorism use can be found in *Medical Management of Biological Casualties Handbook.*[25]

Chapter 1   The Infection Process

When working directly with patients, health care workers risk exposure to pathogens and, if they are susceptible, infection. When receiving treatment in medical facilities, patients can face the same risks. The goal of infection control is to prevent the transmission of pathogens among health care workers and patients. The threat of infection exists in general practices, as well as those specializing in, for example, dentistry, dermatology, podiatry, otolaryngology, ophthalmology, and home health care.

Cycle of Infection

The cycle of infection consists of the five steps shown in Fig. 1. Basic to this cycle is the existence of a pathogen, which may be a bacterium, virus, fungus, or parasitic protozoan. Not all species of these organisms are pathogenic; those capable of producing disease can be:

- <u>Resident</u> pathogens, which normally colonize mucocutaneous body surfaces and cause infection <u>only</u> when introduced into sterile tissues.

- <u>Transient</u> pathogens, which are transmitted to humans and can potentially overcome their defense systems to cause infection.[26,27]

Depending on specific circumstances, some pathogens can be either resident or transient. For example, an immunocompromised, hospitalized patient sneezes into his hand, then rubs his contaminated hand over the intravenous insertion site. The resident nasal *Staphylococcus aureus* becomes transient when it moves to his hand, and could potentially be transmitted to his bloodstream via the immediate contact with nonintact skin, causing an infection.

Reservoirs

Pathogens need reservoirs *(Fig. 1, step 1)* in which to metabolize and reproduce. Depending on the kind of pathogen, a suitable reservoir may be in or on humans, animals, plants, soil, dust, liquids, or food.

When resident pathogens invade normally sterile tissues, they cause endogenous infections.[26] For example, in U.S. hospitals providing acute care, an estimated 3% to 5% of the patients acquire new infections while being treated, but 25% to 50% of these nosocomial infections occur because patients' resident pathogens invade their own sterile body sites when carried by invasive devices[28] (e.g., when health care workers do not properly disinfect the insertion site for a catheter).[29,30]

Exit Vehicles

Transient pathogens are those which escape from an infected or colonized patient or health care worker via exit vehicles *(Fig. 1, step 2)*; they can then invade a susceptible host and cause exogenous infections. Health care workers should consider all body substances, mucous membranes, and nonintact skin potentially infectious until otherwise determined. *(See Standard Precautions in this chapter.)*

Transmission Modes

Pathogens can be transmitted to humans: (1) from other humans; (2) in contaminated air, food, objects, or water; and (3) from infected animals or insects. Airborne, common vehicle, contact, droplet, and vector-borne transmission modes *(Fig. 1, step 3)* are described below.

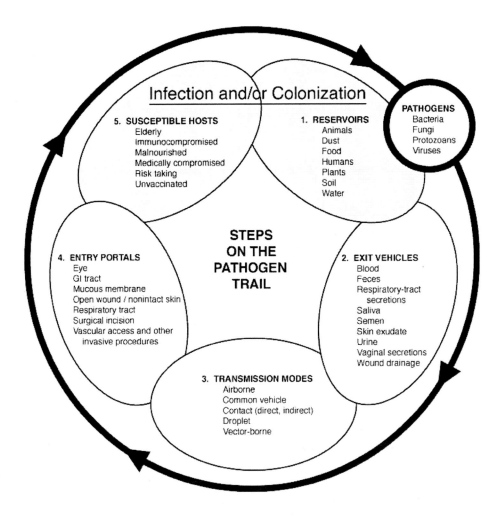

Fig. 1. Cycle of Infection

Airborne transmission. This involves: (1) infectious droplet nuclei (dry particles 5 micrometers or less in size) resulting from evaporation of water in droplets <u>less than 100 micrometers in diameter</u> in respiratory tract secretions of persons infected with, for example, *Mycobacterium tuberculosis;* and (2) contaminated dust particles. Air currents can disseminate suspended droplet nuclei and dust particles distances of more than 3 feet throughout rooms and into other areas of clinics, depending on the type of air handling provided.[1,2,31]

Common vehicle transmission. This involves items often used by more than one person, including: (1) food (e.g., salad bars contaminated with hepatitis A virus, *Shigella sonnei,* or *Salmonella enterica);* (2) water (e.g., contaminated with *Cryptococcus neoformans*); and (3) routine items (e.g., bathroom faucets, doorknobs, or telephone handset grips contaminated with influenza virus). After contact with such items, health care workers must wash their hands before touching patients or themselves (e.g., their eyes, noses, or mouths).

Contact transmission. This can be either direct or indirect:

- Direct contact transmission involves direct body surface to body surface contact, during which pathogens are physically transmitted from an infected or colonized person to a susceptible host.[2] Such transmission can occur, for example, during: (1) patient care activities; (2) childbirth; and (3) open-mouthed kissing[32] and sexual intercourse.

- Indirect contact transmission involves contact between a contaminated intermediate object (e.g., an item in a patient's environment) and a susceptible host.[2] Such pathogen transmission can occur, for example, when: (1) health care workers use contaminated needles, dressings, or instruments for patient treatment, or fail to follow proper handwashing and/or regloving procedures after treating each patient; and (2) people share personal items (e.g., drinking glasses, or toys that children put in their mouths).

Droplet transmission. This involves infectious droplets 100 micrometers or more in diameter in respiratory tract secretions of persons infected with specific pathogens (e.g., influenza viruses and *Neisseria meningitidis).* These large droplets travel distances of less than 3 feet, depending on the means of expulsion; transmission is completed when they reach a recipient's mouth, nasal mucosa, or conjunctivae. However, once droplets fall to the ground, transmission is interrupted.

Vector-borne transmission. This involves contact between a vector (an animal or insect carrying a pathogen acquired from another host) and a susceptible human host. Ticks, fleas, mosquitoes, and rats are often vectors in transmitting pathogens.[2] As an example, mosquito-transmitted West Nile virus infections emerged in the United States during the late 1990s and have since caused many human cases of encephalitis or meningitis and, in some instances, death (e.g., in 2005, 3,000 cases resulting in 119 deaths were reported in the United States).[33]

Entry Portals

Pathogens enter a host through a portal *(Fig. 1, step 4)*. Activities which permit pathogen entry include practicing risky sex, breathing contaminated air, or touching body orifices or cuts with unwashed hands. In health care facilities, surgical incisions and puncture sites (e.g., intravenous insertion or phlebotomy sites) can be portals of entry. Pathogen transmission via contaminated organ transplants and blood transfusions poses a small risk.

Susceptible Hosts

After a pathogen enters a susceptible host *(Fig. 1, step 5)*, it multiplies, and, if it achieves numbers sufficient to overwhelm the host's defense mechanisms, it causes illness.[29] Human defenses include: (1) natural barriers (e.g., intact skin, gastric acid, normal resident bacteria, respiratory tract cilia, and tears); and (2) the immune system (e.g., the inflammatory response and cell-mediated and humoral immunity). The integrity and strength of people's defenses affect their susceptibility to infections; so do environmental factors (e.g., excessively arid air causing mucosal dryness, and contaminated air or equipment).[34] However, the infective potential (infectivity) of pathogens can vary according to each invading species' virulence, toxicity, ability to multiply, and numbers. The route by which pathogens are transmitted and duration of susceptible hosts' exposures can also influence the infection process.

Persons at <u>high risk</u> of becoming hosts include those who:

1. Have chronic illnesses (e.g., asthma, diabetes, obesity, or sickle-cell anemia, or cardiac, pulmonary, renal, or skin diseases).

2. Have undergone intraabdominal, cardiothoracic, or transplant surgery or have an invasive device, such as an indwelling urethral catheter, in place.

3. Are intensive care, long-term care, or burn unit patients, or are neonates.

4. Have diminished immunocompetence, caused, for example, by human immunodeficiency virus (HIV) infection, radiation treatment, chemotherapy, or long-term use of systemic corticosteroids.

Severely immunocompromised persons frequently suffer sepsis syndrome, in which the immune system overreacts to pathogen presence in the blood and releases substances causing deterioration. A 15-month study of sepsis syndrome in eight U.S hospitals showed that patients in intensive-care units accounted for 792 of 1,342 cases.[35] In the United States, about 175,000 people die from sepsis syndrome each year.[36]

Interrupting the Infection Process

Successfully attacking pathogens in human reservoirs to halt the spread of infectious disease has always been difficult. To prevent pathogen transmission from health care worker to patient, patient to health care worker, and patient to patient, workers should routinely:

1. Obtain thorough patient histories. Early recognition, isolation or cohorting, testing, and treatment of infectious persons reduce the spread of infections. Health care workers should also monitor themselves for signs and symptoms of infection.

2. Be vaccinated on a timely basis and encourage their patients to do so *(see Appendix B)*.

3. Follow the mandates of the Occupational Safety and Health Administration (OSHA) bloodborne pathogen final rule *(see Chapters 4 through 10)*.[23]

4. Use two-tier isolation guidelines recommended by the Centers for Disease Control and Prevention (CDC): Tier 1 is called <u>Standard Precautions</u>; Tier 2 is called <u>Transmission-Based Precautions</u>. This chapter describes the basic requirements of these precautions, and

Chapters 2 and 3 indicate which precautions to use when caring for patients with specific infections. Additional recommendations can be found in the CDC 2006 document *Management of Multidrug-Resistant Organisms.*[8]

5. Adhere to work restrictions when infected *(see specific pathogens in Chapters 2 and 3).* The CDC recommends that workers restricted from duty because of job-related exposures or infections not be penalized by loss of wages, benefits, or job status.

6. Receive postexposure prophylaxis *(see specific pathogens in Chapters 2 and 3)* and confidential postexposure medical evaluations *(see Chapter 4)* on a timely basis.

7. Report cases to their facility's designated individual (usually the infection control practitioner), who will in turn report cases to health authorities as mandated by state laws.

8. Perform frequent handwashing or hand antisepsis, and routinely wear personal protective equipment *(see Chapter 5).*

9. Follow published guidelines on sterilizing or disinfecting reusable medical devices and on cleaning the clinical environment *(see Chapters 6 and 7).*

10. Use sharps safely and dispose of them and other regulated waste appropriately *(see Chapter 8).*

Standard Precautions

The CDC has combined the major components of Universal Precautions (which reduce bloodborne pathogen transmission) and Body Substance Isolation (which reduces transmission of all pathogens via any moist body matter) into a single set of infection control guidelines called Standard Precautions.[2] This combination improves protection against pathogen transmission because:

1. Universal Precautions apply to feces, nasal secretions, sputum, tears, urine, and vomitus only when these substances are visibly contaminated with blood. Standard Precautions, however, apply to these substances regardless of whether they contain visible blood, and therefore prevent the transmission of a wider variety of pathogens.

2. Body Substance Isolation does not emphasize handwashing after glove removal unless hands are visibly soiled; Standard Precautions require health care workers to perform hand hygiene immediately whenever they remove gloves.[2]

Standard Precautions—designed to reduce the risk of pathogen transmission from both identified and unidentified sources—apply to: (1) blood; (2) all other body fluids, secretions, and excretions (except sweat); (3) mucous membranes; and (4) nonintact skin.[2] Health care workers must still comply with regulations in OSHA's "Occupational Exposure to Bloodborne Pathogens; Final Rule" (based on the concept of Universal Precautions),[23] but they should go a step further, following the CDC-recommended Standard Precautions, designed to protect both themselves and their patients from infection by any type of pathogen. Algorithm 1 describes the procedures used for Standard Precautions, as well as additional precautions described below.

Transmission-Based Precautions

The CDC restructured its six previous categories of isolation precautions into three—airborne, contact, and droplet—which comprise the new Transmission-Based Precautions. Singularly or in combination, these precautions are to be added to Standard Precautions for patients identified as, or suspected to be, colonized or infected with pathogens known to be transmitted via a specific route.[2] Algorithm 1 describes a few infections against which specific Transmission-Based Precautions are applicable, but Chapters 2 and 3 specify the appropriate precautions to be used against infection with more than 30 pathogens.

Airborne Precautions. These maximum respiratory and isolation precautions are used for patients known or suspected to be infected with pathogens transmitted person to person via droplet nuclei and contaminated dust particles.[2] Health care workers who provide care for patients with active pulmonary or laryngeal tuberculosis must wear personal respirators *(see Chapter 5, Inhalation protection).* Such tuberculosis patients also require use of the special ventilation and air-filtration precautions described in reference 3.

Algorithm 1. Standard and Transmission-Based Precautions

Standard Precautions involve: *	But, if these are added:	Health care workers should also:
• Maintenance of personal hygiene, including appropriate handwashing or hand antisepsis procedures. *(See Chapter 5.)* • Protection against exposure to pathogens, including: 1. Donning gloves just before touching mucosa, nonintact skin, blood, or other potentially infectious materials.** 2. Wearing a surgical mask, eye protection, and protective clothing when splashes of blood or other potentially infectious materials are likely. (See Chapter 5.)	• Airborne Precautions	• Don an N95 or a high-efficiency particulate air (HEPA) personal respirator before entering environments of active tuberculosis patients as protection against infectious droplet nuclei. • Don a surgical mask before entering environments of patients with: 1. Measles (rubeola). 2. Chickenpox (varicella). 3. Disseminated herpes zoster (shingles), or localized herpes zoster that is likely to become disseminated because the patients are immunocompromised.***
	• Droplet Precautions	• Wear a surgical mask when working within 3 feet of patients known or suspected to be infected with pathogens transmitted in large, respiratory tract droplets (e.g., influenza viruses and *Neisseria meningitidis).*
	• Contact Precautions	• Use hand antisepsis. • Don gloves and protective clothing* before entering (and remove these before leaving) environments of patients who are: 1. Infected or colonized with multidrug-resistant pathogens [e.g., methicillin-resistant *Staphylococcus aureus* (MRSA) or vancomycin-resistant enterococci (VRE) or a patient with *Clostridium difficile* diarrhea]. 2. Shedding viruses or bacteria (e.g., diapered patients infected with hepatitis A virus or *Salmonella enterica).*

*   Health care workers should always check with their Infection Control Managers to determine the policies and procedures used in their particular health care facilities.

**   In "Occupational Exposure to Bloodborne Pathogens," OSHA describes "other potentially infectious materials" as: (1) semen and vaginal secretions; (2) amniotic, cerebrospinal, pericardial, peritoneal, pleural, and synovial fluids; (3) saliva in dental procedures; (4) any body fluid that is visibly contaminated with blood; and (5) all body fluids in situations where it is difficult or impossible to differentiate between fluids.[23]

***   Health care workers who are susceptible to measles or chickenpox should, preferably, not be treating patients with these diseases. If they do, they should strictly adhere to recommended precautions: (1) Standard plus Airborne Precautions for measles; and (2) Standard plus Airborne plus Contact Precautions for chickenpox and disseminated herpes zoster.

Airborne Precautions also apply to patients with measles, chickenpox, or certain types of herpes zoster *(see Algorithm 1, Airborne Precautions)*. Workers who provide care for such patients must don surgical masks, and, in hospitals, place the patients in private rooms (preferably kept at negative pressure) with the doors closed. During transport, all of these patients should wear a surgical mask.

Contact Precautions. These reduce the risk of pathogen transmission via skin-to-skin contact (direct contact) and via touching surfaces or patient-care items in a patient's environment (indirect contact). Contact Precautions require that health care workers wear gloves and a gown during <u>any</u> touching or treatment of patients infected or colonized with multidrug-resistant pathogens *(see Algorithm 1, Contact Precautions),* and/or shedding viruses or bacteria in feces or vesicle/lesion secretions. In hospitals, workers should place patients requiring Contact Precautions in private rooms (or cohort them), and limit their transport from the rooms to essential purposes.[2] Workers should also dedicate the use of noncritical-class devices *(see Chapter 7, Low-level disinfection)* to a single patient or a group of patients actively infected or colonized with the same pathogen.

Droplet Precautions. These require health care workers to wear surgical masks when working within 3 feet of (or in the same room or cubicle as) patients known or suspected to be infected with pathogens transmitted in excreted, large, respiratory tract droplets *(see Fig. 2).*

In hospitals, workers should place patients requiring Droplet Precautions in private rooms. If this is not possible, the infected patients should be kept at least 3 feet away from other patients and visitors, and should wear surgical masks when out-of-room transport is necessary.[2]

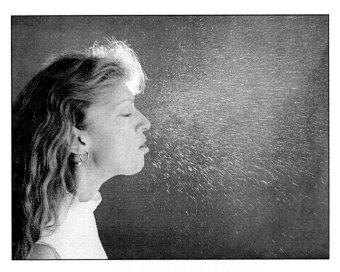

Fig. 2. Hazardous Bioaerosols

One sneeze can produce respiratory tract secretions containing many thousands of infectious droplets. In addition to
using Droplet Precautions themselves, health care workers
should remind their patients to cover their noses and mouths
(if possible, with disposable tissues) when they sneeze or
cough, or to cough or sneeze into their upper sleeve or arm
(not their hands), and to wash their hands afterward.

Chapter Summary

1. Pathogens include many varieties of bacteria, viruses, fungi, and
    parasitic protozoans that infect and/or colonize susceptible hosts.

2. The cycle of infection usually involves five steps:

    Step 1: A reservoir in or on which a pathogen survives.

    Step 2: An exit vehicle by which a pathogen escapes from the
    reservoir.

    Step 3: A transmission mode by which a pathogen travels to a
    susceptible host:

    - Airborne—tiny infectious particles (i.e., droplet nuclei
      or dust) invade a susceptible host's respiratory tract.

- Common vehicle—contaminated, general-use items are used or touched by more than one person.
- Contact:
  - Direct contact—an infectious body surface touches another body surface.
  - Indirect contact—a contaminated object (e.g., unwashed hands) touches or enters a susceptible host.
- Droplet—large infectious droplets in respiratory tract secretions invade a susceptible host's mouth, nasal mucosa, or conjunctivae.
- Vector-borne—an animal or insect carrying a pathogen touches or bites a susceptible human host.

Step 4: A suitable portal of entry, allowing a pathogen to enter a susceptible host.

Step 5: A susceptible host, infected when an invading pathogen multiplies sufficiently to overcome the host's defense mechanisms.

3. Human defense mechanisms include: (1) natural barriers; and (2) the immune system.

4. Standard Precautions apply to: (a) blood; (b) all body fluids, secretions, and excretions (except sweat), regardless of whether they contain visible blood; (c) mucous membranes; and (d) nonintact skin.

5. The three types of Transmission-Based Precautions, used in addition to Standard Precautions when needed, are: (a) Airborne, (b) Contact, and (c) Droplet.

Chapter 2   Overview of Bacteria and Protozoans

This chapter reviews many bacteria and several parasitic protozoans encountered by health care workers in U.S. outpatient practices, hospitals, and nursing homes. Also reviewed are *Bacillus anthracis* and *Clostridium botulinum,* because of their potential for use in biological terrorism activities.

For each pathogen, this chapter describes:

1. The infectious substances involved in the pathogen's transmission and the contagion period.

2. Use of Standard Precautions, plus (if indicated) Transmission-Based Precautions, which reduce the risks of infection for both patients and health care workers.

3. Work practices and personal factors that can increase health care workers' risks of infection. *(See also Chapter 1, Susceptible Hosts.)*

4. Work restrictions that may be imposed on infected workers.

5. Vaccine and postexposure medications (when available) that are recommended for health care workers. *Appendix B provides additional vaccine information (including contraindications and number of doses) for both health care workers and patients.*

6. Case reporting requirements. In clinical settings, health care workers usually report cases to the Infection Control Manager or other designated person, who is responsible for reporting the cases to health authorities.

Bacillus anthracis

Transmission. Environment-to-person transmitted via airborne spore inhalation or contact with contaminated articles. Animal-to-person transmitted via skin contact with infected animals' tissues, contaminated animal products (e.g., hair, wool, hides, and bone meal), and contaminated soil in infected animals' habitats. This Gram-positive bacterium can also be transmitted in undercooked, contaminated meat.[24] Depending on the transmission mode, *Bacillus anthracis* can cause inhalation, cutaneous, oropharyngeal, or gastrointestinal anthrax.

Contagion period. This pathogen is usually not person-to-person transmitted. Rarely it may be transmitted between humans when a person with ungloved hands touches the infected lesions of a person with cutaneous anthrax. *Bacillus anthracis* spores in contaminated soil and materials can remain viable for years.

Recommended precautions. Standard.

Health care worker infection risks. Significant for medical first-responders to anthrax incidents who do not wear full personal protective equipment, including high-efficiency particulate air (HEPA) personal respirators *(see Chapter 5)*. Anthrax-exposed persons should be soap-and-water-decontaminated in a shower.[24]

Work restrictions. Workers with cutaneous anthrax should not provide patient care until their lesions are healed.

Prophylaxis. Unvaccinated laboratory workers exposed to cultures of the bacterium should receive anthrax vaccine *(see Appendix B)*. Unvaccinated health care workers directly exposed to anthrax spores should receive appropriate antibiotics and, if available, the vaccine.[37]

Case reporting. All human cases must be <u>immediately</u> reported to local health authorities, the local Federal Bureau of Investigation office, and the Centers for Disease Control and Prevention (CDC) bioterrorism hotline *(see Appendix A)*.[24]

Bordetella pertussis

Transmission. Person-to-person transmitted in respiratory tract secretions. This Gram-negative bacterium causes pertussis (whooping cough).

Contagion period. From the early catarrhal stage to 3 weeks after onset of paroxysms (e.g., coughing or inspiratory whoop). Patients are usually no longer contagious after 5 days of treatment with antibiotics, but they must complete at least 14 days of the antibiotic regimen to eradicate the bacterium from their upper respiratory tracts and thereby halt its further transmission.[38]

Recommended precautions. Standard plus Droplet.[2] Place hospitalized patients in private rooms (or semiprivate rooms with another pertussis patient) until they have taken erythromycin for at least 5 days.[24]

Health care worker infection risks. Significant for susceptible workers who fail to use appropriate precautions (above) during close, face-to-face contact with patients having, or suspected of having, *Bordetella pertussis* infection.[1] (Killed, whole-cell pertussis vaccines used until the early 1990s provided little or no protection 5 to 10 years after the last dose.)[38]

Work restrictions. Workers with active pertussis must be restricted from duty from the beginning of the catarrhal stage through the third week after onset of paroxysms, or until 5 days after the start of effective antibiotic therapy. Workers who develop unexplained rhinitis or an acute cough following known *Bordetella pertussis* exposure should be restricted from patient care until they have taken erythromycin for 5 days.[1]

Prophylaxis. No vaccine is currently licensed in the United States for persons age 7 or older. Susceptible workers exposed to *Bordetella pertussis* should immediately begin postexposure prophylaxis (a 14-day course of erythromycin or trimethoprim-sulfamethoxazole). Workers exposed to "suspected" pertussis patients whose cultures prove negative and whose clinical courses suggest different diagnoses should discontinue prophylaxis.[38]

Case reporting. In all states, pertussis cases must be reported to local health departments.[24]

Chlamydia pneumoniae

Transmission. Person-to-person transmitted in respiratory tract secretions. This Gram-negative bacterium (previously called Taiwan acute respiratory agent) causes pneumonia.

Contagion period. Prolonged; not well defined.[24]

Recommended precautions. Standard.[2]

Health care worker infection risks. Increased for workers who are immunocompromised or suffer from chronic illnesses, or are cigarette smokers.[39]

Work restrictions. Workers should not provide patient care until acute illness is resolved.

Prophylaxis. No vaccine.

Case reporting. Epidemics of *Chlamydia pneumoniae* infection should be reported to local health departments.[24]

Clostridium botulinum

Transmission. In foods (e.g., those that are inadequately preserved or cooked and, sometimes, honey); also, environment-to-person transmitted in contaminated soil entering wounds. Terrorists could potentially use toxins produced by this Gram-positive anaerobic bacillus as food and drink contaminants and as bioaerosols.[24]

Contagion period. Not person-to-person transmitted.

Recommended precautions. Standard.[2]

Health care worker infection risks. Although person-to-person transmission has not been documented, risks are increased for workers who do not carefully wash their hands after touching soiled diapers of patients with intestinal botulism.

Prophylaxis. No vaccine. Workers who ingest food containing *Clostridium botulinum* and have symptoms of infection should immediately enter an intensive-care unit for management of possible respiratory failure, and be given one vial of polyvalent (AB or ABE) botulinum antitoxin, obtainable from the CDC.[24]

Work restrictions. Workers should not provide patient care until acute illness is resolved.

Case reporting. Most states require reporting of suspected and confirmed botulism cases. However, any case not arising from an obvious contaminated food source should be <u>immediately</u> reported to local health authorities, the local Federal Bureau of Investigation office, and the CDC bioterrorism hotline *(see Appendix A)*.[24]

Clostridium difficile

Transmission. Person-to-person transmitted in feces. Any surface, device, or material (e.g., commode, bathing tub, and electronic rectal thermometer) that becomes contaminated with feces may serve as a reservoir for *Clostridium difficile* spores. The spores are transferred to patients mainly via the hands of health care personnel who have touched a contaminated surface or item.[40]

Contagion period. Duration of diarrhea episodes.

Recommended precautions. Contact Precautions for patients with known or suspected *Clostridium difficile*-associated disease:

- Place these patients in private rooms. If private rooms are not available, these patients can be placed in rooms (cohorted) with other patients with *Clostridium difficile*-associated disease.

- Perform hand hygiene using soap and water to wash spores off hands *(<u>note</u>: no current hand hygiene product kills spores)*; dry hands; then apply an alcohol hand rub.

- Use gloves when entering a patient's room and during patient care.

- Use gowns if soiling of clothes is likely.

- Dedicate equipment whenever possible.

- <u>Continue these precautions until diarrhea ceases</u>.

- Ensure proper cleaning of patient room and environment.

Health care worker infection risks. Limited risk of acquiring symptoms. May become colonized with *Clostridium difficile*. The possibility of developing diarrhea exists if health care workers are taking antibiotics, a major precipitator of the illness.

Work restrictions. Symptomatic health care workers should not provide care until infection is resolved.

Prophylaxis. None.

Case reporting. Outbreaks should be reported to local health departments.

Corynebacterium diphtheriae

Transmission. Person-to-person transmitted in respiratory tract and lesion secretions. This Gram-positive bacterium causes diphtheria.

Contagion period. Until effective antibiotic therapy ends shedding of the bacterium.[24]

Recommended precautions. Standard plus Droplet for patients with pharyngeal diphtheria. Standard plus Contact for patients with cutaneous diphtheria.[2] Infected patients should be placed in private rooms.

Health care worker infection risks. Increased for immunocompromised workers exposed to infected travelers requiring medical care.[1]

Prophylaxis. Health care workers should be vaccinated with tetanus-diphtheria vaccine every 10 years *(see Appendix B)*. Those directly exposed to infected patients' respiratory droplets or cutaneous lesions should have nasopharyngeal cultures taken and be monitored for clinical signs of diphtheria for 7 days. They should also be given antibiotic prophylaxis and one dose of the vaccine if they have not been vaccinated within the previous 5 years. Workers with initial positive cultures should receive antibiotics for as long as they remain culture-positive.[1]

Work restrictions. Exposed workers and those identified as asymptomatic carriers must be restricted from duty until they complete effective antibiotic therapy and have two negative nasopharyngeal cultures obtained at least 24 hours apart.[1]

Case reporting. In most states, diphtheria cases must be reported to local health departments.[24]

Cryptosporidium parvum

Transmission. Person-to-person-transmitted in feces. Also transmitted to humans from contaminated water (chlorination does not kill it), and from infected animals.[24] This enteropathogenic protozoan causes cryptosporidiosis, marked by acute diarrhea.[41]

Contagion period. From illness onset through several weeks after symptoms end, as long as oocysts (the infectious protozoal stage) are shed.[24]

Recommended precautions. Standard. Exception: Standard plus Contact for diapered or incontinent patients.[2]

Health care worker infection risks. Increased for workers who fail to wear gloves during handling of used bedpans or fecally soiled diapers/linens, and fail to wash their hands afterward.[1]

Work restrictions. Workers with acute gastrointestinal symptoms should be restricted from contact with patients and their environments, until their symptoms resolve. They should also consult with local health authorities on work restrictions in their specific locales.[1]

Prophylaxis. None.

Case reporting. All cryptosporidiosis cases should be reported to local health departments.[24]

Escherichia coli Serotype O157:H7

Transmission. Mainly in contaminated foods (e.g., inadequately cooked hamburger and animal feces-contaminated produce or milk); also person-to-person transmitted in feces. Six categories of Gram-negative *Escherichia coli* cause diarrhea; however, serotype O157:H7 can also cause hemorrhagic colitis, hemolytic uremic syndrome, and thrombotic thrombocytopenic purpura.[24]

Contagion period. For as long as the bacterium is shed in feces; this can be as long as 3 weeks in some children.[24]

Recommended precautions. Standard. <u>Exception:</u> Standard <u>plus</u> Contact for diapered or incontinent patients, for duration of illness.[2]

Health care worker infection risks. Increased for workers who fail to wear gloves during handling of used bedpans or fecally soiled diapers/linens, and fail to wash their hands afterward.[1]

Work restrictions. Infected health care workers should not provide care to patients until their symptoms resolve. Employers can consider requiring employees to have two negative fecal samples or rectal swabs that are collected 24 hours apart, but not sooner than 48 hours after they take their last antibiotic dose. Local health authorities should be consulted about requirements for such cultures.[1,24]

Prophylaxis. None.

Case reporting. In many states, *Escherichia coli* infections must be reported to local health departments; however, any groups of bloody diarrhea cases should be reported.[24]

Giardia lamblia

Transmission. Person-to-person-transmitted in feces. This enteropathogenic protozoan causes giardiasis, marked by diarrhea.[42]

Contagion period. As long as the cysts are shed in feces; this can continue for months, especially in infected, immunocompromised persons.[24]

Recommended precautions. Standard. <u>Exception:</u> Standard <u>plus</u> Contact for diapered or incontinent patients.[2]

Health care worker infection risks. Increased for workers who fail to wear gloves during handling of used bedpans or fecally soiled diapers/linens, and fail to wash their hands afterward.[1]

Work restrictions. Workers with acute gastrointestinal symptoms should be restricted from contact with patients and their environments, until their symptoms resolve. They should also consult with local health authorities on work restrictions in their specific locales.[1]

Prophylaxis. None.

Case reporting. In some states, giardiasis cases must be reported to local health departments.[24]

Legionella pneumophila

Transmission. Environment-to-person transmitted, for example, from stagnant hot water in shower heads, faucets, humidifiers, respiratory therapy devices, and whirlpool spas that produce mists.[16] This Gram-negative bacterium causes legionellosis (Legionnaires' disease), a cause of pneumonia.

Contagion period. Not person-to-person transmitted.

Recommended precautions. Standard.[2]

Health care worker infection risks. Increased for workers who are immunocompromised, suffer from chronic illnesses, or are cigarette smokers, if the bacterium is present in water reservoirs in the work environment.[16]

Work restrictions. None.

Prophylaxis. None.

Case reporting. In selected areas, legionellosis cases must be reported to local health departments.[24]

Mycobacterium tuberculosis

Transmission. Person-to-person transmitted mainly in respiratory tract droplets expelled when persons with <u>active</u> tuberculosis of the lung or pharynx cough, sneeze, speak, or sing. Evaporation of the droplets produces infectious droplet nuclei that can bypass upper airway defenses and reach the alveoli (however, the probability of infection depends on the pathogen's concentration in the air, in relation to the volume and rate of air exchanges, and the duration of a person's exposure to it.)[43] Gram-positive *Mycobacterium tuberculosis* can also be transmitted from mothers to fetuses,[44] and from patients with severe lymph node infection and draining tuberculous lesions to an open area in an individual contacting the drainage. Rarely, it is transmitted in blood (e.g., via needlesticks).[45]

Contagion period. Until patients with pulmonary or laryngeal tuberculosis have three consecutive negative sputum tests from sputum collected on different days. [Patients with active tuberculosis of the oral cavity or any part of the respiratory tract, or with draining lesions, are infectious; those with other types of extrapulmonary tuberculosis or whose illness is inactive (latent) are not infectious.][3]

Recommended precautions. Standard plus Airborne [using a high-efficiency particulate air (HEPA), or an N95, personal respirator] for patients with active pulmonary or laryngeal tuberculosis. Exception: Standard only for patients with active extrapulmonary tuberculosis.[2] Health care workers should postpone active tuberculosis patients' elective surgery, dental or ophthalmic exams, and other elective care until presented with physicians' statements confirming that the patients are no longer infectious. *(See Table 1 for additional tuberculosis infection control procedures, including patient isolation.)*[1,3]

Health care worker infection risks. Increased risk for workers: (1) with known exposure to an unidentified, or improperly isolated, infectious tuberculosis patient; (2) involved in prolonged nosocomial tuberculosis outbreaks; and (3) exposed to infectious specimens being processed in laboratories, or infected cadavers being examined in necropsy rooms.[1,46]

Special testing. Workers with potential for exposure to *Mycobacterium tuberculosis* should receive a baseline Mantoux tuberculin skin test; also called the Mantoux purified protein derivative (PPD) test. If they have not had a Mantoux test during the last year and the baseline test is negative, they should be tested again 1 to 3 weeks later. (Infected persons' ability to react to the test diminishes over time; however, if the first test "boosts" the diminished immune response, the second test could be positive, and the second test result should be used as the baseline.)[47] This testing should, preferably, be done before workers are hired or given hospital privileges. Some facilities may use a blood test (QuantiFERON).[3]

Table 1. Tuberculosis Infection Control Checklist	
Precautions	**Health Care Worker Procedures**
Personal respirators.	• When involved in the care of infectious tuberculosis patients, use Standard Precautions <u>plus</u> Airborne Precautions; the latter includes fit-checking and wearing snugly fitting N95 or high-efficiency particulate air (HEPA) personal respirators: 1. Before entering hospital isolation rooms or the homes of such patients, or when transporting the patients. 2. When such patients are undergoing procedures likely to induce coughing, or are coughing (at any time) and will not cover their mouths.
Patient isolation.	• <u>Immediately</u>: (1) separate patients with suspected or active tuberculosis* from others; and (2) give them, and instruct them to wear, surgical masks that fit tightly around their noses and mouths. Then: 1. <u>Dental office workers</u> should quickly arrange for the patients to see physicians or go to hospital emergency rooms for evaluation, thus having them leave the dental-care facility as soon as possible. If the patients need emergency dental care, refer them to a facility with appropriate ventilation and air handling capabilities. 2. <u>Medical office workers</u> should promptly evaluate the patients (ideally, in tuberculosis isolation areas) for possible infectiousness. Medical care settings that provide care to populations at relatively high risk for active tuberculosis should consider use of anti-tuberculosis engineering controls for general-use areas (e.g., waiting rooms). 3. <u>Hospital workers</u> should place infectious patients in tuberculosis negative-pressure isolation rooms. Air is directed into these rooms, then vented to the outside of the building. Germicidal ultraviolet lamps can also be used to kill *Mycobacterium tuberculosis* suspended in droplet nuclei, but short-term exposure to ultraviolet light can cause skin problems, and long-term exposure can increase the risks of skin cancer and cataracts. During transport to and from treatment areas, active tuberculosis patients should wear surgical masks or unvented personal respirators. Details on tuberculosis-prevention engineering criteria, including CDC-recommended hourly room air changes and safeguards against ultraviolet light exposure, appear in *Morbidity and Mortality Weekly Report,* 43 (RR-13), October 28, 1994.

*   When taking patient histories, health care workers should determine whether patients have symptoms suggestive of active tuberculosis (e.g., a cough lasting for 3 weeks or longer, accompanied by night sweats, bloody sputum, fever, or weight loss).

Other recommendations include:

1. Annual skin testing (minimally) for all workers with potential for exposure to the mycobacterium.

2. Semiannual (every 6 months) skin testing (minimally) for workers who are immunocompromised or employed in multidrug-resistant tuberculosis-prevalent areas.

3. Immediate skin testing for workers who did not use Standard <u>plus</u> Airborne Precautions during exposure to active pulmonary or laryngeal tuberculosis; if negative, the test should be repeated 12 weeks later.[1,3] (It can take 2 to 10 weeks after infection for a person to develop an immune response to tuberculin.)[43]

Health care workers who received Bacille Calmette Guérin (BCG) vaccine *(see Prophylaxis)* more than 10 years ago need to be tested; however, those who received BCG within the last 10 years should be individually assessed for the need for testing.[1,3]

Work restrictions. Workers with active pulmonary or laryngeal tuberculosis must be restricted from the workplace until they can provide proof that they are not infectious. Usually, this entails documentation that: (1) they are receiving adequate therapy; (2) their coughs have resolved; and (3) they have had three negative sputum tests on specimens collected on 3 separate days. After resuming work, they must provide periodic documentation that they are remaining on therapy for the recommended period and their sputum test results remain negative.[1,3]

Prophylaxis. Although not recommended as a primary tuberculosis control strategy, BCG vaccination is recommended for health care workers who are employed in areas where multidrug-resistant tuberculosis is prevalent and infection control precautions have failed to prevent transmission of the mycobacterium to such workers *(see Appendix B)*. Prior to receiving the vaccine, workers should consult with local and state health departments, on a case-by-case basis, regarding the advisability of vaccination.[1,43]

Latent tuberculosis. Workers who have positive Mantoux tuberculin skin tests, but negative bacteriologic studies (if done), and no clinical or radiographic evidence of active tuberculosis should receive treatment for latent tuberculosis. This greatly reduces the possibility of activation of their infection in the future. An estimated 10 million to 15 million persons in the United States have noncontagious, latent *Mycobacterium tuberculosis* infection, and, without treatment, about 10% of them will eventually develop contagious, clinically active tuberculosis.[48] For details on drug regimens for specific persons, readers should refer to the *Morbidity and Mortality Weekly Report,* 52(RR-11), June 20, 2003.[49]

Case reporting. All confirmed and suspected tuberculosis cases must be reported to local health departments.[24]

Mycoplasma pneumoniae

Transmission. Person-to-person transmitted in respiratory tract secretions. This Gram-negative bacterium causes pneumonia, especially in children and young adults.

Contagion period. Possibly, from 20 days to 13 weeks.[24]

Recommended precautions. Standard plus Droplet.[2]

Health care worker infection risks. Increased for workers who are immunocompromised or suffer from chronic illnesses, or are cigarette smokers.[39r]

Work restrictions. Workers should not provide patient care until acute illness is resolved.

Prophylaxis. None.

Case reporting. Epidemics of *Mycoplasma pneumoniae* infection must be reported to local health departments.[24]

Neisseria meningitidis (Meningococcus)

Transmission. Person-to-person transmitted in respiratory tract secretions and saliva. Of this Gram-negative bacterium's 13 serogroups, the B, C, and Y serogroups cause most U.S. infections. This bacterium can cause life-threatening meningococcal meningitis and/or fulminant meningococcemia (Waterhouse-Friderichsen syndrome).[18,50]

Contagion period. Until infected patients have completed 24 to 48 hours of effective antibiotic treatment.[24]

Recommended precautions. Standard plus Droplet.[2] Wear a surgical mask until 24 hours after patients start effective antibiotic therapy, and place infected patients in private rooms during this period.[24]

Health care worker infection risks. Increased risks for susceptible workers who: (1) do not wear a mask when providing dental care or performing oropharynx examinations, mouth-to-mouth resuscitation, or endotracheal intubation; or (2) are exposed, in laboratories, to soluble preparations containing the pathogen.[1]

Work restrictions. Infected workers must be restricted from work until 24 hours after they start effective therapy; during this time, they will usually be too ill to work anyway.[1]

Prophylaxis. Health care workers routinely exposed in laboratories to soluble preparations of this bacterium, or working in areas where three or more confirmed or probable serogroup C cases occur during 3 months or less, should receive quadrivalent (A, C, Y, and W-135) vaccine *(see Appendix B)*. Only workers who did not use Standard plus Droplet Precautions while examining an infected patient's oropharynx or performing mouth-to-mouth resuscitation or endotracheal intubation should immediately receive postexposure ceftriaxone intramuscularly, or, if not pregnant, lactating, or taking oral contraceptives, rifampin or ciprofloxacin, orally.[1,18]

Case reporting. All cases of *Neisseria meningitidis* infection must be reported to local health departments.

Salmonella enterica

Transmission. Person-to-person transmitted in feces. Also transmitted in feces-contaminated food and milk.[24] This Gram-negative bacterium causes salmonellosis, marked by acute gastroenteritis.

Contagion period. From infection through several days or possibly weeks. Some infected patients shed *Salmonella* for a year or longer.[24]

Recommended precautions. Standard. Exception: Standard plus Contact for diapered or incontinent infected patients.[2]

Health care worker infection risks. Increased when workers fail to wear gloves during handling of used bedpans or fecally soiled diapers/linens, and fail to wash their hands afterward.[1]

Work restrictions. Infected health care workers should not provide care to patients until their symptoms resolve and they have two consecutive negative stool cultures collected not less than 24 hours apart. However, for workers who have received antibiotics, the first culture specimen should not be taken until 48 hours after the last dose.[24]

Prophylaxis. None for most *Salmonella* species that cause enteric disease.[51] However, workers regularly engaged in research projects on *Salmonella typhi,* which causes typhoid fever, should receive typhoid vaccine.[1]

Case reporting. All salmonellosis cases must be reported to local health departments. Health authorities estimate that about 5 million cases of this disease occur annually in the United States.[24]

Shigella sonnei

Transmission. Person-to-person transmitted in feces during direct physical contact or via touching food, water, or milk with contaminated hands.[24] This Gram-negative bacterium causes shigellosis, marked by acute inflammatory colitis.

Contagion period. From acute infection through about 4 weeks, or as long as bacterial shedding in feces occurs.[24]

Recommended precautions. Standard plus Contact for all diapered or incontinent infected patients.[2]

Health care worker infection risks. Increased when workers fail to wear gloves during handling of used bedpans or fecally soiled diapers/linens, and fail to wash their hands afterward.[1]

Work restrictions. Infected health care workers should not provide care to patients until their symptoms resolve. Employers can consider requiring employees to have two negative fecal samples or rectal swabs that are collected 24 hours apart, but not sooner than 48 hours after they take their last antibiotic dose.[24] Local health authorities should be consulted about requirements for such cultures.[1]

Prophylaxis. None.

Case reporting. In most states, shigellosis cases must be reported to local health departments.[24]

Staphylococcus aureus

Transmission. Person-to-person transmitted, primarily via health care workers' contaminated hands; however, workers carrying the bacterium in their anterior nostrils, axilla, perineum, nasopharynx, or oropharynx may also disseminate it into patients' environments.[1,52] This Gram-positive bacterium causes skin infections, pneumonia, and bacteremia.

Contagion period. As long as infected lesions continue to drain, or persons remain carriers of the bacterium.[24] Under these conditions, infected persons can autoinfect themselves in different body areas.

Recommended precautions. Standard plus Contact if infectious drainage is present—whether it is caused by susceptible or drug-resistant strains [e.g., methicillin-resistant *Staphylococcus aureus* (MRSA) and oxacillin-resistant *Staphylococcus aureus* (ORSA); cases of vancomycin-resistant *Staphylococcus aureus* [VRSA] have recently been reported in the United States). Exception: Standard for patients whose infection does not produce infectious drainage, or who are determined to be colonized (not infected) at a site—whether by susceptible or drug-resistant strains.[2] Use strict handwashing hygiene, and safely dispose of lesion dressings. Current recommendations should be reviewed and adapted to specific health care settings.[8]

Health care worker infection risks. Increased for workers with chronic illnesses or those taking antimetabolites or steroids.[24]

Work restrictions. Health care workers with infected draining lesions should be restricted from patient care, food handling, and any hospital nursery work until they have received adequate therapy and their infections have resolved. Workers suspected to have an infection (versus colonization) should refrain from the above activities until their culture results are negative. Workers with confirmed or suspected carriage of *Staphylococcus aureus* need not have work restrictions unless they are found to be responsible for disseminating the pathogen in health care settings.[1,24]

Prophylaxis. None.

Case reporting. Outbreaks (not individual cases) of *Staphylococcus aureus* infection must be reported to local health departments.[24] Some states have passed legislation that <u>all</u> *Staphylococcus aureus* infections are to be reported to the local health department, and other states are considering such legislation.

Streptococcus pneumoniae (Pneumococcus)

Transmission. Person-to-person transmitted in respiratory tract secretions. This Gram-positive bacterium has 90 known serotypes, but fewer than 25 cause invasive diseases.[53] In addition to persons with clinically active illness, asymptomatic carriers often transmit this bacterium to others.[54] The pneumococcus causes pneumonia, meningitis, bacteremia, and otitis media.[14]

Contagion period. Until patients have completed 48 hours of <u>effective</u> antibiotic therapy.[24] (Because many pneumococcal strains are now penicillin-resistant, third-generation cephalosporins are usually the first-choice drug.)[55]

Recommended precautions. Standard.[2]

Health care worker infection risks. Increased risk for exposed unvaccinated workers who are immunocompromised or chronically ill, or are cigarette smokers.[39]

Work restrictions. None.

Prophylaxis. All health care workers age 65 or older should receive the pneumococcal vaccine. If workers were vaccinated when under age 65, they should be revaccinated at age 65 or older, provided 5 years have elapsed since their primary vaccination. Vaccination is recommended for workers under age 65 if they are immunocompromised or have chronic diseases *(see Appendix B)*.[14]

Case reporting. Epidemics of *Streptococcus pneumoniae* infection must be reported to local health departments.[24] Each year, in the United States, pneumococcal disease accounts for millions of infections.[14]

Streptococcus pyogenes

Transmission. Person-to-person transmitted in respiratory tract secretions, lesion secretions, and pus. Known as group A streptococcus (GAS), the Gram-positive bacterium is also transmitted (rarely) in contaminated milk, deviled hard-boiled eggs, and egg salad.[24] On several occasions, asymptomatic health care workers carrying *Streptococcus pyogenes* have been linked to invasive infections of postoperative and postpartum patients.[56] This bacterium can cause necrotizing fasciitis ("flesh-eating" disease) when wounds it infects are not properly treated; it also causes "strep throat," skin infections (including impetigo), scarlet fever, and illnesses mentioned below.

Contagion period. Until patients have taken penicillin for 24 hours. Untreated carriers can be contagious for 3 weeks or more after infection.[24]

Recommended precautions. Standard <u>plus</u> Droplet for coughing patients whose respiratory tract secretions contain the pathogen. Standard <u>plus</u> Contact for patients producing major lesion secretions and/or pus.[2]

Health care worker infection risks. Increased when workers do not use the above precautions. Following exposure to infected patients' secretions, some health care workers have developed cellulitis, lymphangitis, pharyngitis, or toxic shock-like syndrome[1] (a rapidly progressing illness with a 30% mortality rate).

Work restrictions. Health care workers with *Streptococcus pyogenes*-infected draining lesions should be restricted from patient care or food handling until they have received antibiotic therapy for 24 hours. Workers with confirmed or suspected <u>carriage</u> of *Streptococcus pyogenes* need not have work restrictions unless they are found to be responsible for disseminating the pathogen in health care settings.[1]

Prophylaxis. No vaccine. Antibiotic prophylaxis is recommended only to prevent recurrences of acute rheumatic fever.[57]

Case reporting. Epidemics of *Streptococcus pyogenes* infection must be reported to local health departments. Some locales require reporting of streptococcal toxic shock syndrome and acute rheumatic fever (a potential complication of "strep throat").[24]

Toxoplasma gondii

Transmission. Person-to-person transmitted in utero, or in contaminated transfused blood or transplanted organs.[24] Also transmitted to humans who accidentally ingest cysts in: (1) raw or inadequately cooked meat, or food coming in contact with contaminated meat; (2) dirt containing cat feces; or (3) contaminated soil on unwashed fruits or vegetables.[58,59] This parasitic protozoan causes toxoplasmosis, which, for immunocompetent persons, is usually a mild illness. However, for immunocompromised persons, the infection often invades the brain and causes severe toxoplasmic encephalitis.

Recommended precautions. Standard.[2]

Health care worker infection risks. When female workers are infected during pregnancy, the infection can be transmitted across the placenta to the fetuses. (Children with congenital toxoplasmosis can develop chorioretinitis and intracranial calcifications.)[59]

Work restrictions. None.

Prophylaxis. None.

Case reporting. In some states, *Toxoplasma gondii* infection must be reported to local health authorities.[24]

Vancomycin-Resistant Enterococcus (VRE)

Transmission. Person-to-person transmission, primarily via health care worker contaminated hands and possibly by contaminated equipment (e.g., rectal thermometer probe). Causes urinary tract infections, wound infections, and, sometimes, bacteremias.[8]

Contagion period. As long as infected wounds drain or persons remain carriers (enterococci are normally present in the intestines).

Recommended precautions. Contact Precautions regardless of site of culture (colonization or infection) until three rectal negative cultures a week apart.

Health care worker infection risks. Increased for workers with chronic illness or those immunosuppressed.

Work restrictions. Health care workers with active infection should be restricted until infection resolves.

Prophylaxis. None.

Case reporting. Outbreaks (not individual cases) should be reported to the local health departments.

Chapter Summary

1. The bacteria described in this chapter can be:

    a. Person-to-person transmitted in respiratory tract and lesion secretions, feces, saliva, or blood, or

    b. Environment-to-person transmitted in contaminated food, milk, produce, water, or soil.

2. Most of the protozoans described in this chapter are person-to-person transmitted in feces.

3. Health care workers should always use Standard Precautions; however, when caring for patients with specific bacterial or protozoal illnesses, they should add the following Transmission-Based Precautions.

    a. Airborne Precautions:

        • Active pulmonary or laryngeal tuberculosis.

    b. Droplet Precautions:

        • Pertussis (whooping cough).

        • Pharyngeal diphtheria.

        • Meningococcal meningitis.

        • *Mycoplasma pneumoniae*-caused pneumonia.

        • Respiratory tract *Streptococcus pyogenes* infections that cause patients to cough.

    c. Contact Precautions:

        • *Clostridium difficile*-associated disease.

        • Cutaneous diphtheria.

        • *Staphylococcus aureus* infections if infectious drainage is present, whether it is caused by susceptible or drug-resistant strains.

- *Streptococcus pyogenes* infection with major lesion secretions and/or pus.
- Cryptosporidiosis, giardiasis, salmonellosis, shigellosis, and *Escherichia coli* serotype O157:H7 infections, when patients are diapered or incontinent.
- Vancomycin-resistant enterococcus (VRE) infection regardless of site of culture (colonization or infection)

4. Health care workers should be vaccinated with:

   a. Tetanus-diphtheria vaccine every 10 years.

   b. Meningococcal vaccine, if they are routinely or potentially exposed to *Neisseria meningitidis* in laboratories *(see text)*.

   c. Pneumococcal vaccine, if they are immunocompromised, have chronic diseases, or are age 65 or older. *(See also Appendix B.)*

Chapter 3   Overview of Viruses

This chapter reviews many <u>person-to-person transmitted</u> viruses encountered by health care workers in U.S. health care facilities; also reviewed is the variola virus (the cause of smallpox) because of its potential biological terrorism use. For each virus, the chapter describes items similar to those described for bacteria and protozoans in Chapter 2. Appendix B provides additional vaccine information (including contraindications and number of doses) for both health care workers and patients.

Adenoviruses

Transmission. In respiratory tract and eye secretions. Of the 49 known adenovirus serotypes, about 10 cause most adenovirus-caused outbreaks of acute respiratory disease (including pneumonia) and keratoconjunctivitis.[60] These viruses contain deoxyribonucleic acid (DNA).

Contagion period. For respiratory tract infections, just prior to, and during, clinically active disease. For keratoconjunctivitis, just prior to, and for 14 days after, disease onset, although viral shedding can persist longer.[24]

Recommended precautions. Standard <u>plus</u> Droplet <u>plus</u> Contact for patients with adenovirus-caused pneumonia. Standard <u>plus</u>

Contact for patients with keratoconjunctivitis (includes avoiding hand-to-eye contact).[2]

Health care worker infection risks. Increased for workers who are immunocompromised or suffer from chronic illnesses, or are cigarette smokers.[39]

Work restrictions. Those with keratoconjunctivitis should not be involved in patient care until all their symptoms are gone.[1]

Prophylaxis. None as of 2007. However, in September 2001, the U.S. Army awarded a contract to Barr Laboratories to develop and manufacture adenovirus serotypes 4 and 7 vaccines, which were only available for preventing adult respiratory disease (ARD) among military recruits.[61] (Stocks of these vaccines had been exhausted, after the previous manufacturer ceased production in 1996.)

Case reporting. Epidemics of adenovirus infection should be reported to local health departments.[24] Since 1999, 10% to 12% of all U.S. military recruits have developed adenovirus infection during basic training, and, during 2000, two Navy recruits died from illnesses believed to be caused by adenovirus serotypes 4 and 7.[62] In 1997, a large outbreak of adenovirus serotype 11 infection occurred among civilians at a South Dakota school.[63]

Cytomegalovirus

Transmission. In saliva and urine especially, but also in blood, breast milk, cervical secretions, feces, respiratory tract secretions, semen, and tears.[24] This DNA herpesvirus is known to cause severe retinitis in acquired immunodeficiency syndrome (AIDS) patients and pneumonia in bone-marrow and organ-transplant recipients.

Contagion period. Months to years, as long as the virus is shed, which can occur persistently or episodically.[24]

Recommended precautions. Standard. Use strict handwashing hygiene.[2]

Health care worker infection risks. Because of potential adverse effects of such infection on fetuses, pregnant workers should be counseled on infection control strategies.[1]

Work restrictions. None, if the above precautions are strictly followed.[1]

Prophylaxis. No vaccine. Use of immune globulin and prophylactic antivirals should be considered for noninfected persons who unavoidably receive blood or organs donated by cytomegalovirus-seropositive persons.[24]

Case reporting. Usually not justifiable.[24] In health care institutions, infected young children and immunocompromised patients are the principal cytomegalovirus reservoirs.[1]

Hepatitis A Virus

Transmission. In feces and blood. The primary transmission route is fecal-oral (e.g., putting feces-contaminated food, water, fingers, or other items in the mouth). Rarely, the virus has been transmitted via a blood transfusion.[64] This virus contains ribonucleic acid (RNA).

Contagion period. Two weeks before the onset of jaundice or liver enzyme elevation and during the first week of jaundice. However, young children can shed the virus for several months.[64]

Recommended precautions. Standard. <u>Exception:</u> Standard <u>plus</u> Contact for diapered or incontinent patients.[2]

Health care worker infection risks. Increased when workers fail to wear gloves during handling of used bedpans or fecally soiled diapers/linens, and fail to wash their hands afterward.[1]

Work restrictions. Infected workers should be excluded from patient care areas and food handling for 7 days after symptom onset.[1]

Prophylaxis. Unvaccinated laboratory workers exposed to hepatitis A virus should receive the vaccine *(see Appendix B)*.[64] Unvaccinated health care workers orally exposed to fecal excretions of acute hepatitis A patients should receive one dose intramuscularly of immune globulin as soon as possible (within 2 weeks after exposure). However, the immune globulin is contraindicated for persons who have: (1) immunoglobulin A deficiency; (2) received measles-mumps-rubella vaccine within the previous 2 weeks; and/or (3) received varicella vaccine within the previous 3 weeks.[64]

Case reporting. In all states, hepatitis A cases must be immediately reported to local health departments.[24]

Hepatitis B Virus

Transmission. In blood, blood products, and any body fluids containing visible blood (e.g., bloody saliva, bloody respiratory tract secretions, and menstrual fluids). Blood contains the highest hepatitis B virus titers and is the most common substance in which this DNA virus is transmitted in health care settings. Hepatitis B surface antigen (HBsAg) has also been found in bile, breast milk, cerebrospinal fluid, feces, semen, and synovial fluid; these fluids usually contain low hepatitis B virus titers and, thus, may not be efficient transmission vehicles.[10] However, infected semen passing into the blood, through anal mucosa torn during sexual activity, has frequently transmitted hepatitis B virus infection among male homosexuals.[65]

Contagion period. From many weeks prior to onset of symptoms through acute clinical illness, and, potentially, as long as persons test positive for HBsAg or hepatitis B e-antigen (HBeAg).[24]

Recommended precautions. Standard.[2]

Health care worker infection risks. Highest from needlesticks when source patients' blood is positive for <u>both</u> HBsAg and HBeAg. Unvaccinated workers can also become infected when nonintact skin areas (e.g., cutaneous scratches, abrasions, or burns) or mucosal surfaces are exposed to the virus.[10] Introduction of the vaccine and safety devices has greatly reduced occupational acquisition. Of the 6,104 cases reported to the CDC in 2004, only 75 (1.2%) gave the source as a blood exposure; usually, these individuals either have not started or completed the hepatitis B vaccine series.

Work restrictions. Based on CDC guidelines,[66] individual states have established the circumstances, if any, that restrict health care workers infected with hepatitis B virus from performing exposure-prone invasive procedures (primarily those involving the simultaneous presence of a surgeon's fingers and a sharp object in a poorly visualized or highly confined anatomic site). Infected workers should know their licensing boards' regulations as well.

Prophylaxis. All unvaccinated health care workers at risk of exposure to blood or other body fluids should receive the three-dose series of hepatitis B vaccine *(see Appendix B),* administered in the deltoid muscle. Workers at ongoing risk for blood exposure should be tested 1 to 2 months after they receive all three doses for antibody to HBsAg (anti-HBs). Those failing to show adequate antibody response to the primary vaccine series should repeat it, then be retested, or be evaluated to determine if they are HBsAg-positive.[1] Table 2 describes OSHA-required procedures regarding hepatitis B vaccination.

Table 2. Hepatitis B Vaccine and OSHA Compliance	
Persons	**Responsibilities**
Employers' requirements.	Employers must offer the hepatitis B vaccination series, free of charge, to all employees who risk occupational exposure to blood and other potentially infectious materials.[23] The vaccine must be administered by, or under the supervision of, a licensed health care professional, and employees should receive the first dose within 10 working days of their initial assignments.
Employees' requirements.	Those who decline the vaccination series <u>must</u> sign the following "Hepatitis B Vaccine Declination": "I understand that, due to my occupational exposure to blood or other potentially infectious materials, I may be at risk of acquiring hepatitis B virus infection. I have been given the opportunity to be vaccinated with the hepatitis B vaccine, at no charge to myself. However, I decline hepatitis B vaccination at this time. I understand that, by declining this vaccine, I continue to be at risk of acquiring hepatitis B, a serious disease. If in the future I continue to have occupational exposure to blood or other potentially infectious materials and I want to be vaccinated with hepatitis B vaccine, I can receive the vaccination series at no charge to me." _____ _____ Employee signature Date Provisions governing the initial vaccinations apply if the workers later request them.

Postexposure procedures. The first step following occupational percutaneous, ocular, or mucous membrane exposure to blood or body fluids known, or suspected, to contain HBsAg is <u>immediate first aid</u> *(see Chapter 4).* Then, exposed workers should be evaluated by a knowledgeable health care provider for postexposure prophylaxis, as described in Table 3.

Table 3. Hepatitis B Virus Postexposure Prophylaxis (PEP) Guidelines

If the HCW's immunity status is: *		And the source patient's hepatitis B surface antigen status is:		
Vaccination status	Antibody response	HBsAg-positive	HBsAg-negative	Identity unknown, or unavailable for testing
Unvac-cinated.	—	Recommend HCW PEP: HBIG x 1 and hepatitis B vaccine series.	Recommend HCW PEP: hepatitis B vaccine series.	Recommend HCW PEP: hepatitis B vaccine series.
Previously vaccinated.	Known re-sponder.**	No PEP is recommended.	No PEP is recommended.	No PEP is recommended.
	Known non-responder.[†]	Recommend HCW PEP: HBIG x 1 and revaccination; or HBIG x 2.[††]	No PEP is recommended.	If known to be at high risk for hepatitis B infection, recommend HCW PEP: HBIG x 1 and revaccinat-ion; or HBIG x 2.[††]
	Unknown.	Recommend HCW be tested for anti-HBs. If inade-quate,[†] recommend HBIG x 1 and vaccine booster. If adequate,** no PEP is necessary.	No PEP is recommended.	Recommend HCW be tested for anti-HBs. If inadequate,[†] recommend vaccine booster, and recheck titer in 1 to 2 months. If adequate,** no PEP is necessary.

Abbreviations: anti-HBs = antibody to HBsAg; HBIG = hepatitis B immune globulin; HBsAg = hepatitis B surface antigen; HCW = health care worker.

*   Persons who have previously been infected with hepatitis B virus are immune to reinfection and do not require PEP.

**   A responder is a person with adequate levels of serum antibody to HBsAg (i.e., serum anti-HBs of at least 10 million international units per milliliter).

[†]   A nonresponder is a person with an inadequate vaccination response (i.e., serum anti-HBs of less than 10 million international units per milliliter).

[††] The option of giving one dose of HBIG and reinitiating the vaccine series is preferred for nonresponders who have not completed a second three-dose vaccine series. For persons who previously completed a second vaccine series but failed to respond, two doses of HBIG are preferred. [Table 3 is adapted from Morbidity and Mortality Weekly Report; 50(RR-11).[10]]

When needed, high-titered, hepatitis B immune globulin should be given promptly (i.e., within 24 hours); effectiveness of the immune globulin received more than 7 days after exposure is unknown.[10]

Case reporting. All cases of hepatitis B must be reported to local health departments.[24]

Hepatitis C Virus

Transmission. In blood; currently, hepatitis C virus transmission occurs: (1) mainly, during illicit injecting drug use; and (2) occasionally, during hemodialysis, occupational blood splashes and needlesticks, blood transfusions, and sexual or perinatal exposures.[10,67] Infection with this RNA virus often causes severe, chronic liver disease.

Contagion period. From 1 or more weeks before symptom onset and as long as the patient tests positive for the virus.[24] Many infected persons are asymptomatic for the first 2 decades of the infection and are identified only when they undergo routine biochemical testing or donate blood that is tested for presence of the virus.[67]

Recommended precautions. Standard.[2] In hemodialysis centers, also wear gloves when simply touching patients or hemodialysis equipment, and restrict use of all supplies, instruments, and medications to a single patient.[67]

Health care worker infection risks. Needlesticks with blood-filled, hollow-bore needles pose the greatest risk of occupationally acquired hepatitis C virus infection. Contaminated blood splashes on the conjunctiva also pose risks.[67] Of the 755 cases of acute hepatitis C reported to the CDC in 2004, only 10 (1.3%) were related to new blood exposure.

Work restrictions. None.

Prophylaxis. No vaccine. The first step following occupational exposure to hepatitis C virus is <u>immediate first aid</u> *(see Chapter 4)*. Studies show no support for the use of immune globulin or antiviral agents for postexposure prophylaxis. Following workers' occupational exposures to hepatitis C virus in blood, the source should be tested for antibody to hepatitis C (anti-HCV). If the source is seropositive, the exposed workers should receive baseline testing for anti-HCV and alanine aminotransferase activity, and be retested for such activity 4 to 6 months later. (For earlier diagnosis of possible infection, hepatitis C virus RNA testing can be performed 4 to 6 weeks after the exposure.) Positive enzyme immunoassay anti-HCV results should be confirmed via recombinant immunoblot assay (RIBA™). Seropositive workers should be referred to physicians specializing in treatment of hepatitis C virus infection.[10]

Case reporting. Health care workers should check with local health departments for case reporting requirements. The CDC estimates that 2.7 million persons in the United States have chronic hepatitis C virus infection.[68]

Other Hepatitis Viruses

When caring for patients infected with any of the following viruses, health care workers should use Standard Precautions.

Hepatitis D virus. Transmitted parenterally and sexually, this RNA virus normally infects patients only if their blood contains hepatitis B surface antigen (HBsAg), or they become infected with hepatitis B and D viruses concurrently. The hepatitis B vaccine confers immunity to hepatitis D virus, provided recipients do not already have chronic hepatitis B virus infection.[69]

Hepatitis E virus. Transmitted via the fecal-oral route, this RNA virus most often infects people living in, or having recently visited, certain developing countries. Pregnant patients in the second or third trimester are at high risk (20%) of mortality.[69] No vaccine is available.

Hepatitis G virus. Usually transmitted parenterally, this RNA virus most often infects transfusion recipients, injecting drug (illicit) users, and those already infected with hepatitis C virus.[70] No vaccine is available.

Herpes Simplex Viruses

Transmission. In vesicle fluid, saliva, vaginal secretions, and amniotic fluid.[71] These DNA herpesviruses (types 1 and 2) cause herpes labialis ("cold sores"), herpes genitalis, herpetic whitlow (infection of the fingers), and ocular herpes (often an autoinoculation from an oral outbreak).

Contagion period. Vesicles are infectious from the time they rupture until they are crusted and dry.[71] Intermittent viral shedding from mucosal sites may continue indefinitely.[24]

Recommended precautions. Standard <u>plus</u> Contact.[2]

Health care worker infection risks. Increased for workers who touch herpes simplex virus-contaminated secretions with ungloved hands.[1]

Work restrictions. Workers with herpetic whitlow should be excluded from patient contact until their lesions are healed. Those with orofacial infections should be individually evaluated as to potential transmission of the virus to high-risk patients (e.g., immunocompromised persons, newborns, and children with burns or eczema) and the need for work restrictions.[1]

Prophylaxis. No vaccine. Antivirals may be used to reduce the incidence of recurrent (not primary) infections.

Case reporting. In some states, neonatal herpes simplex infections and/or genital herpes must be reported.[24]

Human Immunodeficiency Virus (HIV)

HIV transmission. In blood, semen, and vaginal secretions. Isolation of HIV from colostrum and breast milk strongly implicates these fluids in cases of postnatal mother-to-infant HIV transmission.[72] This RNA retrovirus causes HIV infection, which in turn causes acquired immunodeficiency syndrome (AIDS).

Contagion period. From immediately after infection to end of life.[24]

Recommended precautions. Standard.[2]

Health care worker infection risks. Increased when workers' percutaneous exposures (e.g., needlesticks) involve a large quantity of HIV-infected blood. This can be: (1) indicated by a device visibly contaminated with the patient's blood, or a deep injury suffered while treating the patient; or (2) associated with placement of a needle directly into a vein or artery, or use of a large-bore hollow needle rather than a solid needle. Workers are also at increased risk during exposure to blood from source patients in the terminal stages of HIV infection/AIDS.[1,10]

Work restrictions. Based on CDC guidelines,[66] individual states have established the circumstances, if any, that restrict HIV-infected health care workers from performing exposure-prone invasive procedures. Infected workers should know their licensing boards' regulations as well.

Prophylaxis. No vaccine. The first step following occupational exposure to blood potentially harboring HIV is <u>immediate first aid</u> *(see Chapter 4).* Then, together with a knowledgeable health care provider, exposed workers should be evaluated for postexposure prophylaxis, as described in Table 4 [adapted from *Morbidity and Mortality Weekly Report,* 54 (RR-09), September 30, 2005]:

- Columns 1 and 2 give guidelines on determining the type and severity or volume of the health care worker's exposure to blood.

- Columns 3 through 7 focus on evaluating the source's HIV status (i.e., using available HIV-status information or performing testing with the source's informed consent or knowledge, depending on specific state laws), or identity (if the source is unknown, assess the epidemiologic likelihood of HIV infection; do not test discarded needles and syringes for HIV contamination).[10]

When postexposure prophylaxis is warranted, a 4-week drug regimen should be initiated, preferably, within 2–4 hours of the exposure.

Expert consultation. Health care workers should call the National Clinicians' Postexposure Prophylaxis Hotline (1-888-448-4911) if :

1. Postexposure prophylaxis is being initiated 24 to 36 hours after the exposure.

2. The exposed health care worker is or is suspected to be pregnant.

3. The source is unknown, or the source's HIV infection is known or suspected to be antiretroviral drug-resistant.

Table 4. HIV Postexposure Prophylaxis (PEP) Guidelines

If the HCW's exposure is:		And the source patient's HIV status* or identity is:			
Type	Severity or volume	HIV+ class 1**	HIV+ class 2***	Status unknown†	Identity unknown††
Percu-taneous	Less severe (e.g., solid needle and superficial injury).	Recommend basic 2-drug PEP.¶	Recommended expanded PEP with 3 or more drugs.¶¶	Generally no PEP warranted; however, consider§ basic 2-drug PEP¶ if source has HIV risk factors.§§	Generally no PEP warranted; consider§ basic 2-drug PEP¶ in settings where exposure to HIV-infected persons is likely.
	More severe (e.g., large-bore hollow needle, deep puncture, visible blood on device, or needle used in patient's artery or vein).	Recommend expanded 3-drug PEP.¶¶	Recommend expanded PEP with 3 or more drugs.¶¶	As above.	As above.
Mucous membrane or nonintact skin§§§	Small volume (a few drops of blood).	Consider basic 2-drug PEP.¶	Recommend basic 2-drug PEP.¶¶	Generally no PEP warranted.§§	Generally no PEP warranted.
	Large volume (a major blood splash).	Recommend basic 2-drug PEP.¶	Recommend expand-ed PEP with 3 or more drugs.¶¶	Generally no PEP warranted; however, consider§ basic 2-drug PEP¶ if source has HIV risk factors.§§	Generally no PEP warranted; consider§ basic 2-drug PEP¶ in settings where exposure to HIV-infected persons is likely.

*   Source: If HIV-negative, no PEP is warranted.

**   Source: HIV positive (+) Class 1—asymptomatic HIV infection or known viral load of fewer than 1,500 HIV RNA copies per milliliter.

***   Source: HIV-positive (+) Class 2—symptomatic HIV infection, AIDS, acute seroconversion, or known high viral load. If drug resistance is a concern, obtain expert consultation: 1-888-448-4911. PEP should not be delayed pending expert consultation; face-to-face counseling, resources for immediate evaluation, and follow-up care for all exposures should be available .

†   Source: HIV status unknown—e.g., a deceased source person with no samples available for HIV testing.

††   Source: identity unknown—e.g., an injury from a contaminated needle in a sharps disposal container or laundry.

¶   Basic 2-drug PEP—see Morbidity and Mortality Weekly Report; 54(RR-09), September 30, 2005.

¶¶   Expanded PEP with 3 or more drugs—see above MMWR.

§   "Consider"—PEP optional, based on an individualized decision between the exposed person and the treating physician.

§§   If PEP is offered and taken and the source is later determined to be HIV-negative, PEP should be discontinued, unless source assessment indicates the possibility of being in the "window period" (recently infected, but not testing HIV-positive as yet).

§§§   Skin exposures—follow up only if there is evidence of compromised skin integrity (e.g., dermatitis, abrasion, or open wound).

Abbreviation: HCW = health care worker.

4. The initial postexposure prophylaxis regimen causes the recipient to suffer adverse symptoms.

5. The exposed individual would benefit emotionally from a second opinion.[10]

Special testing. Regardless of whether postexposure prophylaxis is used, workers occupationally exposed to HIV should: (1) undergo HIV-antibody testing for at least 6 months after exposure (e.g., at baseline, 6 weeks, 12 weeks, and 6 months), or at any time after exposure if they develop an illness compatible with an acute retroviral syndrome; and (2) receive counseling on preventing secondary transmission during the first 6 to 12 weeks after the exposure when most HIV-infected persons are expected to seroconvert.[10]

Case reporting. All states require reporting of new cases of AIDS. The majority of states have surveillance programs requiring providers at confidential HIV testing sites or laboratories performing the tests to report positive results;[24] however, those who report such results should know their states' confidentiality laws.

Influenza Viruses

Transmission. In respiratory tract secretions. These RNA viruses cause influenza A (most severe illness), B (usually milder than type A illness), and C (mild respiratory illness).

Contagion period. The day before symptoms begin through about 5 days after onset.[17] However, children may shed the viruses for 2 weeks.[73]

Recommended precautions. Standard plus Droplet.[2] Place hospitalized patients with confirmed or suspected influenza in private rooms, or, if such rooms are unavailable, in rooms with other influenza patients.[1]

Health care worker infection risks. Infected, unvaccinated workers risk development of pneumonia, especially if they are immunocompromised, pregnant, or chronically ill (e.g., with diabetes), or are cigarette smokers.[39]

Work restrictions. Workers with acute, febrile respiratory infections during community influenza outbreaks should be restricted from care of high-risk patients (e.g., infants and those who are immunocompromised or have chronic obstructive pulmonary disease).[1]

Prophylaxis. All health care workers should receive one dose annually of the current influenza vaccine. Antiviral prophylaxis is not a substitute for influenza vaccination, except for persons for whom the vaccine is contraindicated *(see Appendix B)*. However, antiviral prophylaxis can be used as an adjunct for workers vaccinated after influenza outbreaks have occurred.[17]

Case reporting. Of the influenza viruses, type A causes large epidemics; type B usually causes localized outbreaks; and type C causes only sporadic cases. Cases occurring during epidemics and outbreaks should be reported to local health departments.[24] In recent years, in the United States, influenza outbreaks have caused about 36,000 mortalities annually;[17] however, should an influenza pandemic occur (as, for example, in 1918, 1957, and 1968), many thousands to millions more could die (e.g., H5N1, known as the "bird flu").

Mumps Virus

Transmission. In respiratory tract secretions and saliva. This RNA virus causes mumps, usually marked by painful, enlarged parotid glands.

Contagion period. From 3 days before through 4 days after onset of active disease.[24]

Recommended precautions. Standard plus Droplet.[2]

Health care worker infection risks. Unvaccinated exposed workers can become infected and possibly develop mumps-associated meningitis.[38]

Work restrictions. Workers with active disease must be excluded from duty for 9 days after onset of parotitis. Exposed susceptible workers must be excluded from duty from the 12th day after their first exposure through the 26th day after their last exposure, and/or 9 days after onset of parotitis.[1]

Prophylaxis. All health care workers should be vaccinated against mumps.[11] Although monovalent mumps and bivalent rubella-mumps vaccines are available, the CDC recommends that workers receive trivalent measles-mumps-rubella (MMR) vaccine *(see Appendix B).*[74]

Case reporting. In some states, mumps cases must be reported to local health departments.[24]

Norovirus

Transmission. Transmitted primarily through the fecal-oral route, either by consumption of fecally contaminated food or water or by direct person-to-person spread. Environmental and fomite (i.e., contaminated object or garment) contamination may also act as a source of norovirus infection. Good evidence exists for transmission due to aerosolization of vomitus that presumably results in droplets contaminating surfaces or entering oral mucosa and being swallowed. No evidence suggests that infection occurs through the respiratory system.[75]

Contagion period. During the acute stage of the disease and up to 48 hours after diarrhea subsides.

Recommended precautions. Standard plus Contact if patient is fecally incontinent.[75]

Health care worker infection risks. Increased when glove and hand hygiene protocols are not adhered to.

Work restrictions. Infected health care workers cannot provide care until symptoms subside.

Prophylaxis. None.

Case reporting. Norovirus outbreaks should be reported to local health departments.

Polioviruses

Transmission. In feces, urine, and respiratory tract secretions; also, rarely, in feces-contaminated food, milk, or other items.[1] These RNA enteroviruses (serotypes 1, 2, and 3) cause poliomyelitis, which can be either nonparalytic or paralytic.[19]

Contagion period. For a few days before onset of symptoms and as long as viral shedding occurs (e.g., shedding in feces can last for several weeks to months).[1]

Recommended precautions. Standard.[2]

Health care worker infection risks. Increased for those: (1) working in close contact with patients excreting wild poliovirus (e.g., imported cases); (2) handling specimens containing wild poliovirus; or (3) doing cultures to amplify the virus.[1]

Work restrictions. Workers should not provide patient care until acute illness is resolved.

Prophylaxis. During poliomyelitis outbreaks, previously unvaccinated health care workers occupationally at risk of infection should receive inactivated poliovirus vaccine *(see Appendix B)*. At-risk workers who previously completed the three-dose vaccination series can be given one additional dose.[1,24]

Case reporting. All poliomyelitis cases must be reported to local health departments.[24]

Respiratory Syncytial Virus

Transmission. In respiratory tract secretions. This RNA virus causes bronchial pneumonia and bronchiolitis.

Contagion period. Just prior to, and during, clinically active illness; rarely, infants may shed the virus for several weeks after symptoms disappear.[24]

Recommended precautions. Standard for adolescents and adults with respiratory tract secretions. Standard plus Contact for immunocompromised young children with such secretions.[2]

Health care worker infection risks. Increased when workers: (1) fail to wear masks and protective eyewear when near coughing or sneezing infected patients; and (2) touch their eyes or noses with hands or gloves contaminated with patients' respiratory secretions.[1]

Work restrictions. Workers with acute, febrile respiratory infections during respiratory syncytial virus community outbreaks should be restricted from care of high-risk patients (e.g., infants and those who are immunocompromised or have chronic obstructive pulmonary disease).[1]

Prophylaxis. No vaccine at this time; however, development of one is a high research priority.

Case reporting. Epidemics of respiratory syncytial virus infection should be reported to local health departments.[24]

Rubella Virus

Transmission. In respiratory tract secretions. This RNA virus causes rubella (German measles).

Contagion period. From about 1 week before through at least 4 days after onset of the rash. However, infants born with congenital rubella syndrome may shed large quantities of the virus in their nasopharyngeal secretions and urine for weeks to months.[1,24]

Recommended precautions. Standard plus Droplet for patients infected postnatally. Standard plus Contact for patients with congenital rubella syndrome.[2] Place hospitalized patients in private rooms.

Health care worker infection risks. Unvaccinated, exposed female workers who become infected may develop arthritis, which usually clears within 10 days, but may last for several weeks. Infected pregnant women can transmit the virus to fetuses, possibly causing spontaneous abortion, stillbirth, premature delivery, or congenital malformations.[38,76]

Work restrictions. Workers with active disease must be excluded from duty for 5 days after the rubella rash appears. Exposed susceptible workers must be excluded from duty from the 7th day after their first exposure through 21st day after their last exposure, and/or 5 days after rash onset.[1]

Prophylaxis. All health care workers should be vaccinated against rubella virus; many local and state health departments mandate that such workers be immune to this infection. Although monovalent rubella and bivalent rubella-mumps and measles-rubella vaccines are available, the CDC recommends that workers receive trivalent measles-mumps-rubella (MMR) vaccine *(see Appendix B)*.[74]

Case reporting. All cases of rubella (German measles) and congenital rubella syndrome must be reported to local health departments.[24]

Rubeola Virus

Transmission. In respiratory tract secretions (both large droplets and droplet nuclei). This RNA virus causes measles (rubeola), marked by Koplik's spots on the buccal mucosa early in the disease and a body rash.[38]

Contagion period. From 4 days before through 4 days after rash onset.[24]

Recommended precautions. Standard plus Airborne.[2] Place hospitalized patients in private rooms (preferably kept at negative pressure) with the doors closed, and require them to wear a surgical mask during transport.

Health care worker infection risks. Nonimmune workers should not be caring for patients with measles, which can cause pneumonia, severe laryngotracheitis, and encephalitis.[38] Infected pregnant women can transmit the virus to fetuses, possibly causing aborted pregnancies or premature births.[77]

Work restrictions. Workers with active disease must be excluded from duty for 7 days after the rash appears. Exposed susceptible workers must be excluded from duty from 5th day after their first exposure through the 21st day after their last exposure, and/or 7 days after the rash appears.[1]

Prophylaxis. All health care workers should be vaccinated against rubeola virus; many local or state health departments mandate that such workers be immune to this infection. Although a monovalent measles antigen preparation and bivalent measles-rubella vaccine are available, the CDC recommends that workers receive trivalent measles-mumps-rubella (MMR) vaccine *(see Appendix B).*[74] Susceptible health care workers exposed to rubeola should be vaccinated, within 72 hours after an exposure. Immune globulin, given within 6 days of an exposure, provides only temporary protection (if any) and should be followed by vaccination.[38]

Case reporting. In most states, measles (rubeola) cases must be reported, by telephone or other rapid means, to local health departments.[24]

Varicella Zoster Virus

Transmission. In respiratory tract secretions and vesicle fluid. This DNA herpesvirus initially causes chickenpox (varicella); years later, latent varicella zoster virus-infected cells in ganglia may recrudesce and cause herpes zoster (shingles).[78]

Contagion period. For chickenpox patients, from up to 5 days before the rash appears until all lesions become dried scabs. For herpes zoster patients, until all lesions become dry.[24]

Recommended precautions. Standard plus Airborne plus Contact for chickenpox patients and for herpes zoster patients when the infection is disseminated in any patient, or localized but likely to become disseminated in immunocompromised patients. Exception: Standard only for immunocompetent patients with localized herpes zoster.[2] Place hospitalized chickenpox and disseminated zoster patients in private rooms (preferably kept at negative pressure) with the doors closed, and require them to wear a surgical mask during transport.

Health care worker infection risks. Workers who have not had chickenpox should, preferably, not be caring for patients infected with varicella zoster virus. If they must care for such patients, they need to strictly adhere to the above precautions, which include wearing a gown, a surgical mask, and gloves. If pregnant workers become infected and transmit the virus to fetuses during the first 20 weeks of gestation, newborns may develop congenital varicella syndrome.[38]

Work restrictions. Workers who develop chickenpox or herpes zoster should be excluded from duty until all their lesions dry and crust. Exposed workers should be immediately tested for varicella antibody, even if vaccinated (1% of vaccinees develop mild chickenpox). If negative, the test should be repeated 5 to 6 days later. Workers remaining antibody-negative 7 days following exposure should be excluded from duty in clinical areas where high-risk patients are present, from the 10th day after first exposure through the 21st day after last exposure (28th day if they have received varicella zoster immune globulin).[1,38] In other areas, individual assessments should be made to determine the ability of these workers to work; they can be instructed to immediately report any signs of illness, then be removed from duty.

Prophylaxis. All exposed health care workers lacking reliable chickenpox histories (i.e., documented physician diagnosis or serologic evidence) should receive live attenuated varicella vaccine *(see Appendix B).*[21] Postexposure use of immune globulin is recommended <u>only</u> for immunocompromised or pregnant workers; however, immune globulin is contraindicated for persons who received the varicella vaccine within the previous 3 weeks, unless benefits exceed those of the vaccine.[38]

Case reporting. Many states require chickenpox case reporting, and varicella zoster virus-related deaths should be reported to the CDC.[24]

Variola Virus

Transmission. In respiratory tract secretions. This DNA orthopoxvirus causes smallpox, a disease that was eradicated in the late 1970s; however, terrorists who obtain clandestine variola virus supplies could disseminate them, for example, as bioaerosol clouds.[24]

Contagion period. From appearance of the first lesion through disappearance of all scabs.[24]

Recommended precautions. Standard <u>plus</u> Airborne <u>plus</u> Contact. Patients should be placed in private rooms kept at negative-pressure with the doors closed. However, in the event of a large outbreak, when a sufficient number of negative-pressure rooms are not available, patients can be cohorted and housed in a building (or part of a building) with separate air handling. In such an area, traffic must be restricted, and all persons who must enter the area should adhere to the above precautions.

Health care worker infection risks. Increased for workers who do not use all three recommended types of precautions when caring for patients with smallpox (variola virus infection). Susceptible workers providing care for patients recently vaccinated with vaccinia vaccine risk being infected with this virus if they touch either the vaccination site before the scab separates from the skin, or contaminated bandages covering the site.

Work restrictions. Workers with smallpox must not provide patient care until all their lesions are healed. Those recently vaccinated with vaccinia vaccine should be excluded from duty if they do not keep the vaccination site covered and do not adhere to handwashing practices.[1]

Prophylaxis. Unvaccinated health care workers engaged in research projects on vaccinia virus (the agent used to immunize against smallpox) should be vaccinated every 10 years *(see Appendix B)*.[1] In the event that a case of smallpox is diagnosed, exposed workers should receive the smallpox vaccine within 4 days of exposure.

Case reporting. All cases of smallpox or suspect nonvaricella smallpox-like illnesses must be <u>immediately</u> reported to local health authorities, the local Federal Bureau of Investigation office, and the CDC bioterrorism hotline *(see Appendix A)*.

Chapter Summary

1. The viruses described in this chapter can be person-to-person transmitted in:

   a. Amniotic fluid, blood, breast milk, feces, saliva, semen, tears, and/or urine

   b. Secretions from the eyes, respiratory tract, vagina, lesions, and/or vesicles.

2. Health care workers should always use Standard Precautions; however, when caring for patients with specific viral illnesses, they should add the following Transmission-Based Precautions.

   a. Airborne Precautions:

      • Chickenpox and disseminated herpes zoster (or zoster likely to become disseminated).

      • Measles (rubeola).

      • Smallpox.

    b. Droplet Precautions:

- Adenovirus-caused pneumonia.
- Influenza.
- Mumps.
- Rubella (German measles) in postnatally infected patients.

    c. Contact Precautions:

- Adenovirus-caused pneumonia and/or keratoconjunctivitis.
- Chickenpox and disseminated herpes zoster (or zoster likely to become disseminated).
- Congenital rubella syndrome.
- Herpes simplex virus infection.
- Hepatitis A, when infected patients are diapered or incontinent.
- Norovirus infection, if infected patients are fecally incontinent.
- Respiratory syncytial virus, when infected immunocompromised young children produce respiratory tract secretions.
- Smallpox.

3. Health care workers should be vaccinated with:

    a. Hepatitis A vaccine, if they are exposed to the virus in laboratories.

    b. Hepatitis B vaccine (complete three-dose vaccination series).

    c. Influenza vaccine (annually).

    d. Measles-mumps-rubella (MMR) vaccine, if susceptible to rubeola, mumps, or rubella viral infection.

    e. Inactivated poliovirus vaccine, if occupationally at risk of infection.

    f. Varicella vaccine, if lacking reliable chickenpox histories.

    g. Smallpox vaccine (every 10 years), if performing research on vaccinia virus.

Chapter 4   Occupational Exposure Responses

This chapter reviews responses required by the Occupational Safety and Health Administration (OSHA) and recommended by the Centers for Disease Control and Prevention (CDC) when health care workers are exposed to blood or other potentially infectious materials *(defined in Algorithm 1 footnote).* Such exposures can be:

1. <u>Percutaneous</u>. This type of exposure often results from needlesticks with contaminated hypodermic and butterfly-type needles *(see Chapter 8).* However, during procedures performed with poor visualization, suture needles (blind suturing), bone spicules, and metal fragments can also pose risks to health care workers and patients.

2. <u>Parenteral.</u> Infectious material can be inadvertently injected (e.g., during a needlestick).

3. <u>Mucosal or cutaneous.</u> Blood can enter the eyes, nose, mouth, or nonintact skin via hand transfer, splashes, or sprays (e.g., during irrigation, suctioning, or dental procedures).

Postexposure Responses

Employees occupationally exposed to blood, blood-contaminated body substances, or objects potentially harboring bloodborne pathogens must act quickly to reduce the possibility of infection. They should, in the following order:

1. Use <u>IMMEDIATE</u> first aid.

   a. For a needlestick or cut, or splash on broken skin, wash the skin area with soap and water and/or wipe with alcohol. According to the CDC, there is no evidence that expressing fluid by squeezing the wound or the use of antiseptics for wound care further reduces the risk for human immunodeficiency virus (HIV) transmission; however, antiseptic use is not contraindicated. The CDC does not recommend the application of caustic agents (e.g., bleach) or injection of antiseptics or disinfectants into the wound.[10]

   b. For a splash, spatter, or spray in the eyes, nose, or mouth, flush the exposed mucous membranes with water and/or normal saline. At a minimum, this should be done with tap water from a faucet; <u>preferably</u>, it should be done at an eyewash station, which employers must provide for this purpose *(see Figs. 3 and 4)*.

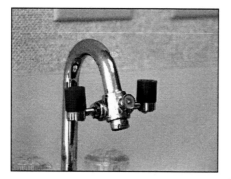   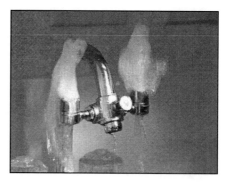

Fig. 3. Eyewash Station Capped   Fig. 4. Eyewash Station Operating

2. Report the incident to your employer or Infection Control Manager, to expedite an evaluation by a licensed health care professional, as described in Table 5.

3. Be evaluated for hepatitis B virus or HIV postexposure prophylaxis *(see Chapter 3, Tables 3 and 4)*, which, if indicated, should begin within 7 days for hepatitis B virus and 2–4 hours for HIV.

OSHA Requirements

Table 5 shows the postexposure evaluation and treatment OSHA requires employers to provide to <u>all</u> employees exposed to bloodborne pathogens.[23] Employees working in states administering their own OSHA-approved occupational safety and health programs *(see Appendix A)* should check the laws regarding employer responsibilities, testing, and confidentiality following an occupational exposure. State health departments can provide information on the locations of their testing sites and those of independent laboratories.

Clinicians evaluating occupationally exposed employees must <u>not</u> reveal blood test results to employers.[23] Some exposure incidents must be resolved through the legal system, particularly when disputes involve the rights of occupationally exposed workers, who test positive for hepatitis B virus or HIV, to receive or administer health care.

Ethical Obligations

When patients are exposed to health care workers' infected blood, such workers have certain <u>ethical</u> obligations. For example, the American Dental Association's (ADA's) *Principles of Ethics and Code of Professional Conduct* states that dentists, regardless of their bloodborne pathogen status, should immediately: (1) inform patients who may have been exposed to blood or other potentially infectious materials in the dental office of the need for postexposure evaluation and follow-up; and (2) refer such patients to a health care practitioner qualified to provide the postexposure services. If dentists are the source individuals, they have ethical obligations to: (1) provide information about their bloodborne pathogen status to the evaluating health care practitioners; and (2) submit to testing that will assist in the patients' evaluations. If the source individuals are staff members or other third persons, dentists should encourage such persons to cooperate as needed for the patients' evaluations.

Table 5. Bloodborne Pathogen Exposures and OSHA Compliance

Requirements for employers:

1. Make immediately available to <u>exposed employees reporting occupational exposure incidents</u>[†] confidential medical evaluations and follow-up, including at least:

   a. Documentation of the exposure routes and circumstances surrounding the incidents.

   b. Source patients' identities (unless employers establish that identification is impossible or prohibited by state/local laws) and blood test results (after exposed employees are informed of laws concerning disclosure of sources' identities and infection statuses). [Source patients' blood can be tested for hepatitis B virus or HIV (if not already known to be infected), immediately after their consent is obtained; employers who cannot obtain legally required consent must establish this fact. Immediate testing of source patients' blood (if available) can be done when consent is not required by law.]

   c. Testing of exposed employees' blood when their consent is obtained. If employees consent to baseline blood collection but do not consent to HIV serologic testing, the samples must be preserved for at least 90 days; if, during this time, the employees elect to have the baseline sample tested, testing must then be done immediately.

   d. Postexposure prophylaxis, when medically indicated.

2. Ensure that all medical evaluations, procedures, and prophylaxis are:

   a. Made available to employees at no cost and at a reasonable time and place.

   b. Performed by or under the supervision of a licensed health care professional.

   c. Provided according to U.S. Public Health Service recommendations applicable when the evaluations and procedures take place.

3. Ensure that all laboratory tests are conducted by an accredited laboratory, at no cost to employees.

4. Ensure that health care professionals evaluating employees occupationally exposed to bloodborne pathogens are provided with:

   a. A copy of OSHA's "Occupational Exposure to Bloodborne Pathogens; Final Rule."

   b. A description of exposed employees' duties as they relate to exposure incidents.

   c. Documentation of the exposure route and circumstances surrounding the exposure.

   d. Results of the source patients' blood testing, if available.

   e. All medical records (including vaccination status) relevant to appropriate treatment of employees; employers <u>must</u> maintain these records *(see Table 27)*.

5. Obtain and provide employees (within 15 days of evaluation completion) with copies of evaluating health care professionals' written opinions, which must be limited to whether:

   a. Hepatitis B vaccinations are indicated for employees and if employees have received such vaccinations.

   b. Employees have been informed of the evaluation results and any medical conditions resulting from occupational exposure that require further evaluation or treatment. *All other findings or diagnoses must remain confidential and cannot be included in the written report.*

[†] According to OSHA, occupational exposure is a reasonably anticipated skin, eye, mucous membrane, or parenteral contact with blood or other potentially infectious materials that may result from the performance of an employee's duties. OSHA uses the same term to describe an actual occupational exposure incident.

Chapter 5 At-Work Personal Infection Control

To protect themselves and their patients, health care workers must practice at-work personal infection control in compliance with Occupational Safety and Health Administration (OSHA) requirements, and should also adhere to Centers for Disease Control and Prevention (CDC) and Association for Professionals in Infection Control and Epidemiology (APIC) guidelines.

Handwashing and Hand Antisepsis

Frequent, thorough handwashing is the most important step in preventing pathogen transmission in hospitals and clinical practices. Cross-contamination occurs when health care workers' inadequately washed hands spread pathogens from: (1) one patient to another; (2) patients to health care workers; and (3) health care workers to patients.[28] Self-infection can occur when health care workers touch their eyes, noses, or mouths with contaminated hands. Table 6 shows OSHA handwashing requirements.[23]

Adhering to Standard Precautions, as well as Standard plus Contact Precautions *(see Algorithm 1),* requires that health care workers use appropriate handwashing or hand antisepsis procedures.

Table 6. Handwashing and OSHA Compliance	
Persons	**Responsibilities**
Employers' requirements.	1. Provide employees with readily accessible handwashing facilities (an adequate supply of running potable water, soap, and single-use towels or hot-air drying machines). 2. Ensure that employees wash their hands immediately or as soon as possible after removal of gloves or other personal protective equipment. 3. Ensure that employees wash skin with soap and water or flush mucous membranes with water immediately following contact of such body areas with blood or other potentially infectious materials. *(See also Chapter 4.)* 4. Provide—when handwashing facilities are not feasible—either an appropriate antiseptic hand cleanser in conjunction with clean cloth/paper towels, or antiseptic towelettes.
Employees' requirements.	1. Wash hands as described in items 2 and 3 above. 2. After washing hands as described in item 4 above, also wash hands with soap and running water as soon as possible.

The CDC strongly recommends that health care workers wash their hands thoroughly with either plain (nonantimicrobial) or antimicrobial soap, if visibly dirty or contaminated with proteinaceous material, or if visibly soiled with blood or other body fluids.[7] If hands are <u>not</u> visibly soiled, health care workers can use an alcohol-based hand rub (alternatively, wash hands with an antimicrobial soap and water) in the following clinical situations:

1. Before and after each patient contact [patient contact includes having contact with anything in the patient's room (e.g., bed rails, bedside table)].

2. After touching blood, body fluids, secretions, excretions, and contaminated items, regardless of whether gloves are worn.

3. After removing gloves or other personal protective equipment.

4. Before donning sterile gloves when inserting a central intravascular catheter.

5. Before inserting indwelling urinary catheters, peripheral vascular catheters, or other invasive devices that do not require a surgical procedure.

6. Between tasks on a single patient, as needed, to prevent transferring pathogens from an infected or colonized site to a noninfected site.[2,7]

Hand-Cleansing Methods and Agents

The choice of hand-cleansing method and agent depends, in general, on the degree of hand contamination, the type of patient care being rendered, and patients' susceptibility to infections.[27] However, health care workers should know the specific recommendations of their health care facilities' Infection Control Managers.

Routine Handwashing

This type of handwashing can be used: (1) to remove soil (e.g., blood or feces) prior to hand antisepsis; (2) before and after eating or using the bathroom; (3) after coughing or sneezing; and (4) after mucosal/substance contact causing low-level microbial hand contamination. Routine handwashing involves:

1. Wetting hands with running water, and applying plain (nonantimicrobial) soap.

2. Rubbing <u>all</u> hand surfaces (i.e., between each finger and the forefinger and thumb; and the front and the back of each hand) vigorously for at least 10 to 15 seconds, or longer if hands are visibly soiled. *(Rubbing generates friction that dislodges pathogens from the skin.)*

3. Rinsing hands thoroughly under running, cool-to-lukewarm water (repeated exposure to hot water may increase the risk of dermatitis).[7]

4. Drying hands thoroughly with disposable towels, covering any breaks in the skin with sterile dressings, and gloving.[27] *[Health care workers do not have to glove if they have no nonintact skin on their hands <u>and</u> they will have contact with <u>only</u> intact skin and noninfectious body substances (e.g., sweat) of patients.]*

Fingernails. Health care workers should keep their fingernails short to reduce debris collection; the CDC recommends keeping natural fingernail tips less than 1/4-inch long).[7] Artificial fingernails/extenders are contraindicated for direct caregivers. Health care workers should also gently remove debris from under their fingernails, using a rounded plastic or orange-wood stick under running water.[7]

Hand Antisepsis

Table 7 describes steps for hand antisepsis.[2,27] Examples of activities requiring use of hand antisepsis include:

1. When <u>both</u> Standard and Contact Precautions must be used [e.g., for patients with *Clostridium difficile* diarrhea, perform routine handwashing *(above)* to wash off spores, dry hands, then use an alcohol hand rub].

2. Before and after touching nonintact skin.

3. Before caring for children who have viral infections or diarrhea.

4. Before caring for high-risk patients and those infected with drug-resistant pathogens.

5. After touching potentially contaminated objects.[2]

Surgical Hand Scrub

Table 7 describes steps for the surgical hand scrub. This scrub is required before performing surgical procedures and when caring for patients in locations where a scrub is required (e.g., surgical ward or special care nursery).[7,27] The CDC recommends that health care workers remove rings, watches, and bracelets before beginning the surgical hand scrub.[7]

Hand-Cleansing Products

Soap dispensers. Soap should not be added to a partially empty soap dispenser. The practice of "topping off" dispensers can lead to bacterial decontamination of soap. Employers should ensure that dispensers function adequately and deliver an appropriate volume of the product.[7]

Dermatitis. When frequent use of an agent causes dermatitis, health care workers should consult with their Infection Control Managers or Employee Health Office about using a milder handwashing or hand antisepsis agent until their skin heals.

Table 7. Hand Antisepsis and Surgical Hand Scrub Steps	
Hand Antisepsis	**Surgical Hand Scrub**
Using a liquid antimicrobial soap:	**Using a liquid antimicrobial soap:**
1. Wet hands with running water.	1. Wet hands with running water.
2. Press antimicrobial soap dispenser release with a paper towel and apply 3 to 5 milliliters of the agent to hands.	2. Apply 3 to 5 milliliters of antimicrobial agent (usually chlorhexidine or iodophor) on hands and forearms.
3. Rub <u>all</u> hand surfaces vigorously for at least 10 to 15 seconds. *(Longer than 15 seconds may be required for visibly soiled hands.)*	3. Generate friction, using a soft sterile brush or disposable sponge, on <u>all</u> hand surfaces for the length of time recommended by the manufacturer, usually 2 to 6 minutes. *(Health care workers should consult with their Infection Control Managers.)*
4. Rinse hands thoroughly under running, cool-to-lukewarm water. *(For sinks without an automatic shutoff or foot control, use a clean paper towel to shut off the faucet.)*	4. Rinse thoroughly under running, cool-to-lukewarm water. *(Keep hands higher than the elbows, and rinse from the fingertips to the elbows.)*
5. Dry hands with disposable towels.	5. Dry one hand, then the forearm with a sterile towel. *(Use a separate, sterile towel to dry the other hand and forearm.)*[7,27]
Using an alcohol-based hand rub:	**Using an alcohol-based hand rub with persistent activity:**
1. Wash visible soil from hands with nonantimicrobial soap and water. *[Not required when hands are not visibly soiled and brief routine activities (e.g., taking blood pressure or handing objects to patients) are being carried out with noncontagious patients.]*	1. Pre-wash hands and forearms with a nonantimicrobial soap; then dry them completely.
2. Dry hands <u>thoroughly.</u>	2. Apply the hand rub to all surfaces of hands and forearms, according to the manufacturer's instructions.
3. Apply hand rub to palm of one hand and rub hands together, covering <u>all</u> hand and finger surfaces until they are dry. Follow manufacturer's instructions on volume of product to use.[7]	3. Allow hands and forearms to dry thoroughly before donning sterile gloves.[7]
	In the surgical setting, use of alcohol-based preparations is usually reserved for health care workers who are sensitive to antimicrobial agents.

Employers should provide personnel with efficacious hand-hygiene products that have low irritancy potential, particularly when these products are used multiple times per shift (i.e., products used for hand antisepsis before and after patient care in clinical areas and those used for surgical hand scrub).[7] The CDC also recommends that employers solicit employees' input regarding the feel, fragrance, and skin tolerance of any products under consideration.

Hand lotions. Hand lotions used in the workplace should be approved by Infection Control Managers to: (1) assure their compatibility with antimicrobial agents; and (2) identify when they should be used. Health care workers should also use hand lotion when off duty.

Antimicrobial agents. Table 8 shows the characteristics of five antimicrobial agents in hand-cleansing products used in U.S. health care settings.[27]

Personal Protective Equipment

Because differing procedures are performed in specific health care settings, the types of personal protective equipment required also differ. OSHA requires employers to:

1. Assess their workplaces for hazards necessitating personal protective equipment use, and record the assessment.

2. Train employees in proper use of such equipment *(see Chapter 9, Table 26).*

3. Fulfill all requirements shown in Table 9.[23,79]

OSHA considers personal protective equipment adequate if it prevents blood or other potentially infectious materials from reaching employees' work clothes, street clothes, undergarments, skin, or mucosa (e.g., oral or conjunctival), under normal conditions of use and for the entire time the personal protective equipment is used.

Protective Gloves

Gloves are an adjunct to, not a substitute for, handwashing.[15] Health care workers who do not routinely wear disposable (single use only) gloves *(see Table 11)* risk pathogen invasion through any tiny breaks in the skin on their hands. Workers should remove and dispose of their gloves, wash their hands, and reglove:

Table 8. Antimicrobial Agents in Hand-Cleansing Products			
Ingredient	**Activity**	**Faults**	**Comments**
Alcohols: ethyl (ethanol), isopropyl, or normal-propyl (*n*-propyl)—60% to 90%.	• Bactericidal (most vegetative Gram-negative and Gram-positive species including mycobacteria). • Virucidal (only for in vitro studies). • Fungicidal.	• Not sporicidal. • Ineffective for removing soil (e.g., blood or feces). • Ineffective in alcohol-impregnated wipes (insufficient alcohol content). • Cause skin roughness unless product contains emollients.	Reduces skin microbial counts rapidly.
Chlorhexidine gluconate—4% in a detergent base, or 0.5% chlorhexidine gluconate combined with 70% isopropyl.	• Bactericidal (Gram-positive species <u>except</u> mycobacteria). • Virucidal (only for in vitro studies).	• Less effective against Gram-negative bacteria than Gram-positive bacteria; minimal activity against mycobacteria and fungi. • Affected by differences in skin pH, secretions, and moisture levels.	Remains active on skin for at least 6 hours.
Iodophors—7.5% povidone-iodine formulation for surgical hand scrub.	• Bactericidal (Gram-positive and Gram-negative species). • Virucidal. • Fungicidal.	• Rapidly neutralized in the presence of organic materials. • Possible skin absorption and irritation.	Acts against a wide range of pathogens.
Parachloro-metaxylenol—0.5% to 3.75%.	• Bactericidal (Gram-positive species <u>except</u> mycobacteria).	• Only fair activity against Gram-negative bacteria, mycobacteria, viruses, and some fungi.	Remains active on skin for a few hours.
Triclosan—1% concentration to reduce methicillin-resistant *Staphylococcus aureus* colonization.	• Bactericidal (Gram-positive species and most Gram-negative species).	• Ineffective against fungi. • Activity against viruses is unknown.	Is persistently active on skin.

1. Between caring for different patients. *(Do not wear the same pair of gloves for the care of more than one patient, and do not wash gloves between uses with different patients.)*

Table 9. Personal Protective Equipment and OSHA Compliance	
Persons	**Responsibilities**
Employers' general personal protective equipment requirements.	1. Provide employees at risk of occupational exposure to blood or other potentially infectious materials with free, appropriate, personal protective equipment such as, but not limited to, gloves, gowns, laboratory coats, face masks, eye protection, and ventilation devices including mouthpieces, resuscitation bags, and pocket masks.
	2. Ensure that personal protective equipment is available in appropriate sizes for all employees.
	3. Ensure that employees use appropriate personal protective equipment. (Under extraordinary circumstances, employees might temporarily and briefly decline to use the personal protective equipment because they believe its use would impede the delivery of health care or public safety services or would pose an increased hazard to their safety or that of a coworker. When employees have made this judgment, employers must investigate and document the circumstances, to determine whether changes can be instituted to prevent such occurrences in the future.)
	4. Provide cleaning, laundering, repair, replacement, and disposal of required personal protective equipment at no cost to employees.
Employees' requirements.	1. Remove all personal protective equipment before leaving work.
	2. Place it in a designated area or container for storage, washing, decontamination, or disposal. Items which do not fit OSHA's definition of "regulated waste" *(see Chapter 8)* can be disposed of as ordinary trash, provided state and local laws do not mandate otherwise.

2. Between caring for different body sites on the same patient.

3. On a predetermined basis during lengthy procedures.

4. When glove integrity is compromised or in doubt.[7,27,80]

Table 10 shows OSHA requirements for the use of gloves.[23]

Glove use tips. Health care workers also should:

1. Inspect their gloves, before donning them, for defects such as pinholes, cracks, water stains, or mold; do not use defective gloves. *(To prevent deterioration of new gloves, store them in a cool, dry place where they are not exposed to ultraviolet light, heat, ozone, and/or water.)*

2. Keep their fingernails short enough so they will not tear gloves; avoid wearing jewelry for the same reason.

Table 10. Gloves and OSHA Compliance	
Persons	**Responsibilities**
Employers' requirements.	1. Fulfill general personal protective equipment requirements in Table 9. 2. Provide, for employees allergic to standard gloves, hypoallergenic gloves or glove liners, powderless gloves, or other alternatives.
Employees' requirements.	1. Wear gloves when: a. Having hand contact with blood, other potentially infectious materials, mucosa, and/or nonintact skin. b. Performing vascular access procedures. c. Handling or touching contaminated items or surfaces. 2. Replace disposable (single-use) surgical or examination gloves as soon as possible when they are contaminated, torn, or punctured. (Disposable gloves must not be washed or decontaminated for reuse.) 3. Discard utility gloves if they are cracked, peeling, torn, punctured, or exhibit other signs of deterioration. If their integrity is not compromised, utility gloves can be reused after health care workers: (1) wash them with soap and water while wearing them, or (2) remove them and wash them after donning examination gloves.

3. Avoid stretching gloves excessively, when donning them, and make sure they fit snugly but not too tightly.

4. Remove torn or punctured gloves immediately, peeling them off (turning them inside out) so contamination does not contact their skin; then, drop the gloves directly in the regulated waste container, wash and dry their hands, and reglove.

Handwashing following glove removal is vital because hands can become contaminated during glove removal and when fluids penetrate gloves through: (1) perforations caused by sharp instruments or devices used during clinical care; and/or (2) manufacturing defects (i.e., 1.4% to 6% of new gloves have invisible holes).[81] Also, while gloves are being worn, resident and transient pathogens can multiply in the warm, moist environment inside gloves.

Types of gloves. Table 11 shows three types of gloves used by health care workers;[82] choice depends on the specific tasks to be performed. No gloves are totally impervious to punctures or tears.

Table 11. Gloves Used in Health Care Settings		
Types	**Characteristics**	**Comments**
Examination.	• Nonsterile or sterile, disposable (single use only). • Natural rubber latex,[†] vinyl, nitrile, thermoplastic elastomers, polyethylene, or polyurethane. • Kept in original, dated box until donned. • Available as anatomically correct left- and right-handed pairs.	• Choose nonsterile gloves for most nonsurgical patient care. (If powdered[†] gloves are used, thoroughly remove residual powder from the surfaces of the gloves after donning them.) • Choose sterile examination gloves for treating severely immunocompromised patients (nonsterile gloves can carry fungal spores which can become airborne and invade such patients' respiratory tracts).
Surgical.	• Sterile, disposable (single use only). • Natural rubber latex,[†] chloroprene, or thermoplastic elastomers. • Kept in unopened package until donned.	• Choose surgical gloves for procedures involving surgical entry into tissues, cavities, or organs, or repair of major traumatic injuries. (If powdered[†] gloves are used, thoroughly remove residual powder with a sterile sponge/towel after donning them.)
Utility.	• Nonsterile. • Washable and reusable (provided integrity is not compromised). • Heavy latex[†] or nitrile.	• Choose utility gloves when sterilizing instruments, disinfecting equipment, or cleaning the clinical environment. (These nonmedical gloves <u>cannot</u> be used for tasks involving patient contact.)

[†] Because of health care workers' potential allergic reactions to latex, the National Institute for Occupational Safety and Health recommends that only <u>reduced protein, powder-free latex gloves</u> be worn, and, when performing tasks not likely to involve pathogen contact (e.g., food preparation, routine housekeeping, or maintenance), health care workers wear <u>nonlatex gloves</u>.[83]

Studies also show that double-gloving for surgical procedures results in fewer inner-glove perforations, providing added protection for both surgery personnel and their patients.[84,85]

Latex hypersensitivities. Health care workers' increased use of latex gloves has produced more reports of sensitization to proteins in natural rubber latex. The proteins can: (1) leach out from gloves when exposed to wearers' perspiration; and/or (2) adhere to cornstarch glove lubricant, then become airborne (as latex protein-cornstarch) when powdered gloves are donned or removed.[86]

Localized rashes following latex glove use often result from manufacturing-process additives (e.g., accelerators to vulcanize rubber and antioxidants to prolong glove life). Among health care workers, factors linked to latex sensitization include: (1) frequency and/or duration of latex glove use; (2) elevated total immunoglobulin E levels; and (3) the presence of other allergic conditions (e.g., asthma, eczema, hay fever, or allergic responses to eating bananas, avocados, pears, or chestnuts).[1] Certain patients (e.g., those with urogenital anomalies or who have had multiple operations) become sensitized to natural rubber latex proteins, following frequent exposure to health care workers' gloves and other latex-containing health care items.[87] Algorithm 2 explains two types of allergic reactions to latex.[1,86,87]

Algorithm 2. Allergic Reactions to Natural Rubber Latex			
If, after exposure to latex, you have:	**Which developed:**	**Consider the possibility of:**	**Which, if confirmed by your physician, means you should:**
Asthma, allergic conjunctivitis, hives, nasal pruritis, rhinitis, wheezing, or systemic anaphylaxis.	Shortly after either: • Direct tissue or mucosal contact with natural rubber latex, or • Inhalation of airborne latex-laden cornstarch particles.	Contact urticaria syndrome, a Type I allergic reaction.	• Avoid the use of all latex products,[†] because mild symptoms can progress to severe, systemic reactions and even death. • Carry an allergy alert card and injectable epinephrine for emergency use, if Type I allergic reaction is confirmed.
A delayed, localized rash.	24 to 72 hours after exposure to substances added to gloves during their manufacture.	Allergic contact dermatitis, a Type IV allergic reaction.	• Use nonlatex gloves or gloves labeled "hypoallergenic" (the latter prevent reactions to manufacturing-process additives, but not to proteins in natural rubber latex).

[†]   Health care workers who suspect they have a mild latex allergy should use nonlatex gloves or cautiously try powder-free, reduced-protein latex gloves, or double-gloving with cloth or vinyl gloves beneath latex gloves.

To avoid further exposing at-risk patients to latex, health care workers should, during history-taking, ask them whether they have allergic responses (e.g., itching, a rash, or wheezing) to eating the above-mentioned foods or using latex products such as utility gloves, condoms, and toy balloons.

OSHA-Required Inhalation and Eye Protection

During dental, surgical, laboratory, and postmortem procedures, health care workers are routinely exposed to pathogen-containing spray, spatter, splashes, and/or droplets. Exposure can also occur during suctioning, intubation, bronchoscopy, endoscopy, and cleaning of instruments used for these and other procedures.[80] Table 12 describes inhalation and eye protection required by OSHA for all such procedures.[23]

Table 12. Masks and Eye Protection—OSHA Compliance	
Persons	**Responsibilities**
Employers' requirements .	Fulfill OSHA's general personal protective equipment requirements described in Table 9.
Employees' requirements .	Wear masks in combination with eye protection devices (i.e., goggles or eyeglasses with solid side shields or chin-length face shields) whenever splashes, spray, spatter, or droplets of blood or other potentially infectious materials *(defined in Algorithm 1 footnote)* may be generated, with probable eye, nose, or mouth contamination.

Types of Inhalation Protection

Surgical masks. These cup-shaped or flat, disposable masks do not provide respiratory protection against droplet nuclei containing *Mycobacterium tuberculosis*, because they lack a tight face seal and do not allow fit-testing.[88,89] Surgical masks, when secured tightly, can be used to fulfill OSHA bloodborne pathogen requirements *(see Table 12),* and as protection against chickenpox, measles, and all infections requiring Droplet Precautions. Health care workers should remove and properly dispose of these masks after caring for each patient and when they become moist with exhaled air (which decreases filtering efficiency).

Personal respirators. Both the N95 (N category at 95% efficiency) particulate respirator and the high-efficiency particulate air (HEPA) respirator are National Institute for Occupational Safety and Health (NIOSH)-certified as protection against droplet nuclei produced by tuberculosis patients. *(See Figs. 5 and 6.)* The N95 has a 95% bacterial filtration efficiency (BFE) for particles as small as 0.3 micron, and the HEPA has a 95% BFE for particles as small as 1 micron.[90,91] (The N95's "N category" means "not resistant to oil aerosols," since these are rarely encountered in health care settings; if they are present, an oil-proof respirator is available.)

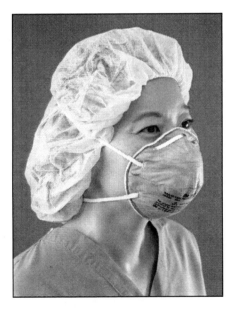

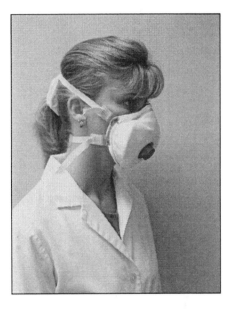

Fig. 5. N95 Particulate Respirator and Surgical Mask

This model of the N95 protects wearers against droplet nuclei <u>and</u> patients against 99% of wearer-generated pathogens. *Photo: courtesy of 3M Health Care.*

Fig. 6. Vented HEPA Respirator

The center exhalation valve enhances wearer comfort, but it also allows the health care worker's secretions to exit, prohibiting use of the respirator during surgical procedures when patients must be protected from all pathogens.

Fit-testing and fit-checking. Both the N95 and HEPA personal respirators must be capable of being:

1. Reliably fit-tested to verify a face-seal leakage of no more than 10%. (When air enters through gaps in the face-to-faceplate seal, the respirator provides virtually no protection against infectious droplet nuclei.)

2. Fit-checked, in two ways, each time they are donned:

   a. Negative fit-check. The wearer covers the respirator's filter surface and inhales. If properly sealed, the respirator will adhere firmly to the face, due to negative pressure created inside the respirator.

   b. Positive fit-check. The wearer exhales. The respirator should lift slightly off the face to allow air to escape around the seal. (If the respirator has an exhalation valve, it must be covered during this fit-check.)[90]

Eyeglasses, goggles, or beards must not be allowed to interfere with face seal integrity. Various models of respirators are being marketed, and fit-testing must be redone each time employees start using a different model (e.g., when employers change brands or employees change jobs).

Algorithm 3 summarizes uses of masks and personal respirators in health care settings, according to the types of precautions involved. OSHA requires that employers provide cleaning, disinfection, and inspection for required reusable respirators *(see Table 9)*; damaged or inefficient HEPA or N95 respirators must be discarded. When not actually in use, neither masks nor personal respirators should be worn around the neck.

Ventilation devices. OSHA also requires employers to provide ventilation devices (e.g., mouthpieces, resuscitation bags, and pocket masks) as alternatives to mouth-to-mouth resuscitation, for use when employees, including emergency response personnel, risk exposure to blood or other body fluids.[23] Disposable resuscitation equipment and devices may be used only once; reusable devices should be disinfected after each patient, according to manufacturers' recommendations.

Algorithm 3. Masks and N95 or HEPA Personal Respirators		
When using:	Wear a:	As protection against:
Standard Precautions.	• Single-use surgical mask.	• Blood and other potentially infectious materials, as required by OSHA *(see Table 12).*
Standard plus Droplet Precautions.	• Single-use surgical mask.	• Respiratory tract secretions (large droplets) produced by patients with, e.g., influenza, mumps, rubella, pertussis, and meningococcal infection. The mask should be worn when working within 3 feet of such patients, unless specific practice rules require workers to don it before entering the patients' rooms.
Standard plus Airborne Precautions.	• Personal respirator (N95, or HEPA*).	• Respiratory tract secretions (droplet nuclei resulting from droplet water evaporation) produced by patients with known or suspected active pulmonary or laryngeal tuberculosis.
	• Single-use surgical mask.	• Respiratory tract secretions (droplet nuclei or large droplets) produced by patients with measles or chickenpox.

* HEPA = high-efficiency particulate air.

Types of Eye protection

When procedures might expose health care workers' facial mucosa to blood or other potentially infectious materials, OSHA requires that eye protection (i.e., goggles or eyeglasses with solid side shields) be worn <u>in combination with</u> masks or respirators *(see Table 12).* Face shields worn as eye protection must fit close against the wearers' foreheads. Even though face shields are chin length, health care workers must wear masks with them because, during procedures generating blood or other potentially infectious materials, pathogen-filled splashes, spray, or spatter can get underneath them. Patients should also be provided with eye protection when needed (e.g., when dental procedures could produce bloody spatter).

Accidental exposure response. If infectious substances do splash, spatter, or spray in an employee's eyes (or nose or mouth), the affected area must be flushed with water <u>immediately</u> *(see Chapter 4, Figs. 3 and 4 showing an eyewash station).*

Eyewear cleaning. OSHA requires that employers provide cleaning for protective eyewear at no cost to employees. Visibly soiled eyewear must be <u>disinfected</u> before being used during treatment of another patient.

Special Dentistry Barriers

Dental professionals can further reduce their eye, nose, and mouth mucosal exposure to infectious bloody spatter or salivary mists by:

1. Placing a rubber dam, when appropriate, on the patient's teeth prior to using handpieces.

2. Using high-volume evacuation during ultrasonic, air turbine, and air-polishing procedures.

Some studies have shown that a preprocedural antimicrobial rinse can reduce the level of oral microorganisms generated during routine dental treatment; however, the scientific evidence remains inconclusive as to whether such rinses actually <u>prevent</u> clinical infections.[9,92,93]

Protective Clothing

The types and characteristics of protective clothing depend on the degree of exposure anticipated.[94] Only long-sleeved, high-necked, fluid-proof or -resistant outer garments (often disposable) prevent patients' body fluids from coming in contact with health care workers' skin and personal clothing.[80,95]

Table 13 shows OSHA requirements for protective clothing, as well as processing of laundry. Health care workers should remove their protective clothing after each patient (before leaving the patient's environment, taking care not to contaminate remaining garments).[2] When outer garments are penetrated by infectious substances, they should be removed immediately, without contaminating the wearer's face or head; pullovers can be cut off with scissors.

After placing contaminated garments in a designated area or container, workers should immediately wash their hands and any other skin surfaces that may have been exposed to infectious substances.[23] Employees should not launder their protective clothing at home; these garments must be laundered either in the clinic or by a laundry service.[95]

Table 13. Protective Clothing, Laundry, and OSHA Compliance	
Persons	**Responsibilities**
Employers' requirements.	**Clothing:** • Fulfill personal protective equipment general requirements in Table 9. **Laundry:** • Provide laundering of reusable protective clothing at no cost to their employees. • Ensure that employees who have contact with contaminated laundry wear protective gloves and other appropriate personal protective equipment. • Ensure that wet contaminated laundry is placed and transported in leakproof bags or containers. • Ensure that laundry bags or containers are labeled or color-coded *(see Chapter 8, Table 24)*. Health care facilities which comply with Universal Precautions in the handling of all soiled laundry can use alternative labeling or color-coding, if all employees will recognize the containers as requiring such compliance. Laundry-filled bags or containers shipped to facilities <u>not</u> using Universal Precautions in the handling of all laundry must be properly labeled or color-coded.
Employees' requirements.	**Clothing:** • Wear appropriate protective clothing such as, but not limited to, gowns, aprons, lab coats, clinic jackets, or similar outer garments, in situations which involve occupational exposure to blood or other potentially infectious materials. • Wear surgical caps or hoods and shoe covers or boots in instances when gross contamination can reasonably be anticipated (e.g., autopsies or orthopedic surgery). • Remove immediately, or as soon as possible, all garments visibly penetrated by blood or other potentially infectious materials. **Laundry:** • Minimize handling and agitation of contaminated laundry. • Sort or rinse laundry only in areas designated for that purpose.

Other Personal Infection Control

OSHA prohibits eating, drinking, smoking, handling of contact lenses, and applying cosmetics or lip balm in work areas where there is a risk of exposure to bloodborne pathogens. Health care workers must <u>not</u> keep food and drinks in refrigerators, freezers, or cabinets, or on shelves, countertops, or benchtops holding potentially infectious materials. Mouth pipetting/suctioning of blood or other potentially infectious materials is prohibited.[23]

Chapter Summary

1. Inadequate handwashing in health care settings spreads pathogens from one patient to another, from patients to health care workers, and from health care workers to patients.
2. Health care workers must choose whether to use routine handwashing, hand antisepsis, or surgical hand scrub, according to the foreseeable degree of hand contamination, type of patient care being rendered, and patients' susceptibility to infection.
3. Antimicrobial agents can be bactericidal, virucidal, fungicidal, or any combination of these. All have certain disadvantages, and must be selected with care.
4. Protective gloves are an adjunct to, <u>not</u> a substitute for, handwashing.
5. Because of health care workers' potential allergic reactions to latex, the National Institute for Occupational Safety and Health (NIOSH) recommends that only <u>reduced protein, powder-free latex gloves</u> be worn, and, when performing tasks not likely to involve pathogen contact, health care workers wear <u>nonlatex gloves</u>.
6. Masks and eye protection devices guard health care workers from blood and other potentially infectious materials; personal respirators protect health care workers from droplet nuclei containing *Mycobacterium tuberculosis*.
7. The degree of exposure anticipated determines the choice of protective clothing. Employers are responsible for providing employees' reusable protective clothing and laundering of it.

Chapter 6   Sterilizing Instruments

Sterilization is the use of a physical or chemical procedure to destroy all forms of microbes on medical and surgical instruments and devices.[23] This chapter reviews basic sterilization procedures, including Occupational Safety and Health Administration (OSHA) requirements and Centers for Disease Control and Prevention (CDC) and American Dental Association (ADA) recommendations. When possible, health care workers should use single-use, disposable instruments (sterile when purchased), so they can discard pathogens instead of having to kill or inactivate them. (Unlike sterilization, disinfection—discussed in Chapter 7—eliminates many but not all forms of microbes.)

Susceptibility of Microbes

Some pathogens are more difficult to destroy than are others. Examples, according to their resistance to heat or chemicals, include:

1. Most difficult to kill: prions that cause kuru and Creutzfeldt-Jakob disease in humans *(see Table 15 footnote)* and the thick-walled endospores of bacteria (e.g., *Bacillus anthracis* and *Clostridium botulinum*).

2. Slightly less difficult to kill: mycobacteria (e.g., *Mycobacterium tuberculosis),* hydrophilic or nonlipid viruses (e.g., poliovirus and rhinovirus), fungi (e.g., *Candida albicans* and *Cryptococcus*

neoformans), and vegetative bacteria (e.g., *Staphylococcus aureus* and *Salmonella enterica).*

3. <u>Least difficult to kill:</u> lipophilic or lipid viruses (e.g., hepatitis B virus and human immunodeficiency virus); <u>however</u>, even these require stringent sterilization measures.[96,97]

Instrument Classifications

As described in Table 14, all medical instruments and devices classified as critical and most of those classified as semicritical must be <u>sterilized</u> after each patient.[96,98,99,100] Chapter 7 describes disinfection of semicritical devices (when appropriate) and noncritical devices.

Sterilants and Their Uses

Before using sterilants, health care workers must:

1. Read the manufacturers' instructions (and warranties) for all chemicals and equipment to be used, to protect both themselves and the equipment.

2. Ask their Infection Control Managers about their health care facility's sterilization policies.

3. Know applicable local, state, and federal regulations on medical instrument processing.

Table 15 shows the characteristics of several sterilants in current use.[92,98,101,102,103,104,105,106] Factors affecting decisions on which sterilants are appropriate include: (1) the class of instrument or device to be sterilized; and (2) the item's tolerance of heat, moisture, or strong chemicals.

<u>Vital to the success of the sterilization process is health care workers' detailed knowledge of manufacturers' instructions for:</u>

1. Loading, operating, and monitoring sterilizers.

2. Use of Food and Drug Administration (FDA)-approved liquid sterilants, formerly approved by the Environmental Protection Agency (EPA).

Table 14. Critical- and Semicritical-Class Instruments or Devices			
Classes	**Examples of Items**		**Required Sterilization**[†]
Critical: items that penetrate soft tissue, bone, or the vascular system, or allow blood to flow through them.	• Arthroscopes. • Bone chisels. • Cardiac catheters. • Cystoscopes. • Forceps. • Implants. • Laparoscopes.	• Needles • Periodontal scalers, metal and nonmetal. • Scalpels. • Surgical and dental burs. • Ultrasonic scaler tips.	High-temperature sterilization, or, if items are heat-intolerant, exposure to other types of sterilants described in Table 15.
Semicritical: Items that do not meet critical-class criteria, but <u>do</u> contact either mucous membranes or broken skin.	• Air/water syringe tips. • Amalgam condensers. • Bronchoscopes. • Cryosurgical instruments. • Diaphragm-fitting rings. • Endoscopes	• High-speed handpieces. • Laryngoscopes. • Low-speed handpiece intraoral components. • Oral mirrors. • Plastic film holders. • Rag wheels. • Vaginal speculums.	Sterilization, or, if items cannot tolerate heat or long exposure to liquid sterilants, high-level disinfection (*described in Chapter 7*). Clean and heat sterilize dental handpieces and intraoral instruments that can be removed from air and water lines of dental units between patients.

[†] The American Dental Association recommends that <u>all</u> reusable, critical- and semicritical-class dental instruments be heat- or gas-sterilized. Dental health care workers can refer to the ADA's detailed list of sterilization methods for specific items.[92] Some states mandate that high-speed handpieces be sterilized after each patient; currently produced high-speed handpieces are heat-tolerant; earlier models must be either retrofitted with heat-stable components or discarded.[100]

"Flash" sterilization, in which sterilizers are operated at much higher than usual temperatures, for shorter periods, should be used only in emergency situations (e.g., when an instrument in short supply is dropped on the floor in an operating room).[107] This method should not be used for implantable devices.[108]

Dry Heat

Dry heat in static-air and forced-air ovens offers the advantage of not corroding predried instruments containing carbon steel. In a static-air oven, the heat rising from coils in the bottom of the chamber transfers its energy to the instruments. A forced-air sterilizer circulates hot air rapidly throughout the chamber.[95]

Table 15. Sterilants and Characteristics of Their Use

Types of Sterilants	Required Temperatures or Times*	Characteristics of Sterilants
Dry heat: static air.	• 1 hour; 340°F (171°C). • 2 hours; 320°F (160°C).	• **Positive:** (1) can be biologically monitored; (2) penetrates closed containers; and (3) is noncorrosive for predried items. • **Negative:** (1) does not penetrate organic debris; (2) does not sterilize liquids; and (3) can damage plastic and rubber.
Dry heat: forced air.	• Packaged items, 12 minutes; 375°F (190°C). • Unpackaged items, 6 minutes; 375°F (190°C).	• **Positive:** (1) can be biologically monitored; (2) penetrates closed containers; and (3) is noncorrosive for predried items. • **Negative:** (1) does not penetrate organic debris; (2) does not sterilize liquids; and (3) can damage plastic, rubber, some metals, and soldered joints.
Ethylene oxide (EtO) gas.	• 10 to 16 hours; unheated unit, at room temperatures of 67°F (19°C) to 75°F (24°C). • 2 to 3 hours; heated unit, 120°F (49°C).	• **Positive:** can be biologically monitored. • **Negative:** (1) does not penetrate aluminum foil; (2) can be explosive in the presence of sparks or flames; (3) leaves noxious gas in rubber and plastic items not sufficiently aerated (e.g., unheated units require 24 or more hours of aeration; heated units, 8 to 12 hours); and (4) requires proper ventilation (i.e., OSHA limits EtO vapor level to 1 part per million average over 8 hours).
Glutaraldehyde.	• 10 hours exposure time; room temperatures of 68°F (20°C) to 77°F (25°C).	• **Positive:** is generally noncorrosive. • **Negative:** (1) cannot be biologically monitored; (2) prohibits packaging of instruments; (3) becomes ineffective with dilution and repeated use; and (4) requires proper ventilation (i.e., 10 air exchanges per hour in air-conditioned rooms); vapor levels greater than 0.1 part per million can irritate eyes, nose, and throat.
Hydrogen peroxide.	• 74 minutes; room temperature of about 68°F (20°C), for Sterrad® 100 sterilizer.	• **Positive:** (1) can be biologically monitored; and (2) allows packaging of instruments. • **Negative:** (1) cannot be used for critical or semi-critical dental instruments, implants, flexible endoscopes, linens, cellulosics, liquids, or powders.

* Does not include unit warm-up time or, for ethylene oxide, aeration time. Consult manufacturers' recommendations for warm-up, exposure, and aeration times, <u>all of which depend on</u> the size and composition of a load and the type of unit.

Table 15 (Continued). Sterilants and Characteristics of Their Use		
Types of Sterilants	**Required Temperatures or Times***	**Characteristics of Sterilants**
Peracetic acid.	• 12 minutes exposure time during overall cycle of about 25 to 30 minutes; 122°F (50°C) to 132°F (56°C).	• **Positive:** can be biologically monitored, although efficacy has been questioned. • **Negative:** (1) cannot be used for critical or semicritical dental instruments; (2) prohibits packaging of instruments; (3) can be used only once, with one processor *(see text);* and (4) can corrode brass, bronze, copper, galvanized iron, and plain steel (but additives can reduce corrosion).
Steam.	• 15 to 40 minutes; 250°F (121°C). *Except for the Creutzfeldt-Jakob disease prion.* **	• **Positive:** (1) can be biologically monitored; and (2) can sterilize water-based liquids. • **Negative:** (1) does not penetrate closed containers or aluminum foil, or reliably penetrate oils, fats, greases, powders, or glass-syringe tight interstices; (2) can dull cutting edges; (3) can damage plastic and rubber; (4) can corrode carbon steel (using 2% sodium nitrite spray or dip may inhibit corrosion); and (5) produces mercury vapors in amalgam-containing extracted teeth.
Unsaturated chemical vapor.	• 20 to 30 minutes; 270°F (132°C).	• **Positive:** (1) can be biologically monitored; and (2) is usually noncorrosive for predried items. • **Negative:** (1) does not penetrate aluminum foil, fabric, or closed containers; (2) does not sterilize liquids; (3) becomes ineffective as chemicals evaporate; (4) can damage plastic and rubber; and (5) requires proper ventilation (OSHA limits formaldehyde exposure to 0.75 part per million average over 8 hours).

*   Does not include unit warm-up time. Consult manufacturers' recommendations for warm-up, exposure, and aeration times, <u>all of which depend on</u> the size and composition of a load and the type of unit.

** For medical and surgical instruments/devices contaminated with the Creutzfeldt-Jakob disease prion, processing time is at least 30 minutes at 270°F (132°C) in gravity displacement autoclaves, and 18 minutes at 273°F (134°C) to 281°F (138°C) in vacuum displacement autoclaves.

Ordinary kitchen and table-top ovens are <u>not</u> Food and Drug Administration-approved for use as sterilizers.[101]

Ethylene Oxide

Hospitals often use ethylene oxide (EtO) to sterilize instruments, equipment, and materials that would be damaged by high temperatures. To avoid potential explosion and fire, manufacturers mix ethylene oxide with 90% carbon dioxide (an ethylene oxide-freon mixture was used prior to government restrictions on use of freon). Ethylene oxide sterilizers have two components: a sterilizing chamber and an aeration cabinet. Exposure and aeration times are shorter for heated units than for unheated units.[102,108] Compact units are available for use in small clinical practices.

Glutaraldehydes

These sterilant solutions should be used only on instruments or devices that cannot tolerate high temperatures. The Food and Drug Administration has approved at least 10 brands of glutaraldehydes;[109] none of these kills all bacterial endospores unless items are meticulously precleaned, rinsed, and dried, then completely submerged in the chemicals for <u>10 hours</u> at manufacturer-recommended temperatures (failing to meet these criteria, the process produces disinfection, <u>not</u> sterilization).[95,96,108,110]

Hydrogen Peroxide

Many U.S. hospitals use the large Sterrad® 100 Sterilizer.[109,111,112] The hydrogen peroxide plasma sterilization process involves five consecutive stages in the chamber: (1) a vacuum is drawn; (2) 58% hydrogen peroxide solution is injected; (3) hydrogen peroxide vapor is diffused for 50 minutes; (4) radio frequency energy generates a plasma field for 15 minutes; and (5) HEPA-filtered air is introduced, to return atmospheric pressure to the chamber.[113] In the plasma field, the hydrogen peroxide vapor breaks apart into free radicals, which collide/react with and kill microbes.[105] A smaller unit, the Sterrad® 50, uses two vapor-diffusion plasma stages and requires only a 45-minute cycle time.[114]

Peracetic Acid

The Food and Drug Administration has approved a peracetic acid sterilant, restricting the product to one-time-use with the tabletop Steris

System 1™ Processor.[109] This processor mixes prefiltered water with a packaged concentrate of 35% peracetic acid, diluting it to a final concentration of 0.2%; rinsing and air drying of sterilized items are automatic. Although biological monitoring of the sterilization cycle is possible, the idea of performing such monitoring in a liquid has yet to gain widespread acceptance among infection control experts (e.g., they question whether agitation would release the endospore strips, clamped within the sterilizing chamber, into the solution).[106,115]

Steam

Steam autoclaving *(Fig. 7)* penetrates pathogenic organic debris, paper wrappings, and fabric more efficiently than other heat sterilization methods.

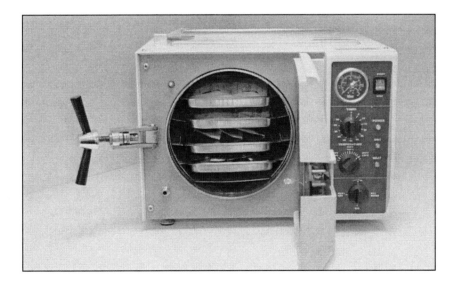

Fig. 7. Steam Autoclave

Instrument packages contain chemical indicators that change color in response to temperature inside the sterilizer chamber. Use of perforated shelves and porous wrappers or containers improves steam penetration.

Autoclaves are either: (1) the gravity displacement type, in which entering steam forces the cooler, denser air out of the chamber through the autoclave drain; or (2) the vacuum displacement type, in which air is removed from the chamber before steam enters it (this type achieves better steam penetration of wrapped and porous items).[103,108] When lubricating instruments to be autoclaved, health care workers should: (1) use a water-based lubricant which allows the steam to penetrate and sterilize all instrument parts; and (2) remove excess lubricant from the instruments.[116]

Unsaturated Chemical Vapor

The efficiency of chemical vapor sterilizers depends on synergism of the chemicals used (e.g., some manufacturers recommend a solution of formaldehyde, alcohol, ketones, acetone, and water). The solution must be monitored to ensure proper levels of alcohol and ketones, because these chemicals evaporate more with each sterilization cycle.[101] Units equipped with a purge system, which collects chemicals from the vapors inside the chamber, produce less odor when the unit door is opened.[95]

Sterilization Steps

Health care workers must first determine which sterilization methods manufacturers recommend as safest and most effective for specific instruments and devices. Then, health care workers should:

1. Don personal protective equipment (i.e., utility gloves, mask, eyewear, and protective clothing); wear it during tasks requiring handling of contaminated instruments.

2. Complete all six basic steps described below (as applicable). Omission of any step could compromise the integrity of instruments or devices.

Presoaking Instruments (Step 1)

Table 16 describes presoaking procedures for instruments that cannot be cleaned immediately after use.[95,107,117] Presoaking dissolves or softens debris on the instruments, making later cleaning easier and more effective. The contaminated presoaking solution should be discarded at least once a day, more often if it appears soiled.

Table 16. Presoaking Procedures
1. Wipe gross blood and tissue off the instruments. *(For reusable sharps, use a one-handed technique; see Chapter 8.)*
2. Place the instruments in a portable basket submerged in cold water,[†] containing soap or a detergent-disinfectant labeled for instrument submersion; do <u>not</u> use hot water, which coagulates blood and protein, for pre<u>soaking</u> purposes.
3. Let the instruments soak for no longer than a few hours, to avoid corrosion of instruments containing carbon steel.
4. Drain the presoaking solution. According to the CDC, liquid waste may be poured carefully into a drain connected to a sanitary sewer system,[100] but check local and state regulations first. *(See also Chapter 8, Liquid Waste.)*
5. Rinse the instruments thoroughly in the basket, using tap water and avoiding water splash.

[†] <u>Exception</u>: For dental handpieces, wipe off visible debris; then, with bur in chuck, flush the handpieces by operating them with water for 30 seconds, aimed into a running high-velocity evacuation system, or a dry throw-away towel. This removes any contamination that may have gotten into the lines. Then, remove the handpieces from hoses and thoroughly clean, rinse, and dry their exteriors.

Precleaning Instruments (Step 2)

The CDC advises the use of a <u>covered</u> ultrasonic cleaner *(see Fig. 8 for uncovered view),* rather than manual scrubbing, for precleaning (the removal of all foreign material from instruments).

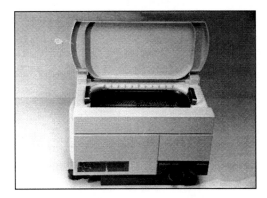

Fig. 8. Ultrasonic Cleaner

Use of this equipment for precleaning increases efficiency, eliminates pathogenic spray, and minimizes handling of sharp instruments.

Ultrasonic cleaner procedures. The energy in an ultrasonic cleaner produces billions of bubbles in the cleaning solution. Collapsing bubbles create turbulence which dislodges debris from the surface of the instruments.[95,100]

Table 17 describes the procedures for efficient precleaning, a process which <u>must</u> precede effective sterilization.[92,95,96,107,118]

Table 17. Precleaning Procedures

1. Place the rinsed, presoaked, or just-used instruments in an ultrasonic cleaner basket or cassette rack.

2. Put the container into the ultrasonic cleaner;[†] make sure the cleaning solution completely covers the instruments.

3. Cover the machine tightly to prevent escape of contaminated airborne pathogens.

4. Process the instruments until they are visibly clean. (This usually takes 10 to 15 minutes, but the time varies with different machines, so follow the manufacturers' instructions. Instruments in plastic or resin cassettes require longer processing because the cassettes absorb some of the ultrasonic energy.)

5. Remove the instrument-laden basket or rack and rinse it thoroughly under tap water, minimizing splash.

6. Using forceps, separate and remove instruments from the basket/rack. (OSHA prohibits hand removal of contaminated sharp instruments from a container.)

7. Inspect instruments for any remaining debris and remove it carefully (e.g., dental cement or wax may have to be removed with solvents).

8. Dry the instruments thoroughly; lubricate them, if necessary, using a water-based lubricant.

[†] <u>Exception:</u> When manufacturers do <u>not</u> recommend ultrasonic cleaning for their dental handpieces, spray a cleaner or, if needed, a cleaner/lubricant into the assembled handpiece,[92] and expel (with bur in chuck) excess cleaner and lubricant into a vacuum line, handpiece cover, or gauze pad. To preclean fiberoptic handpieces, clean the fiberoptic connecting interfaces according to manufacturers' instructions.[107]

Only eight to 10 loose instruments should be ultrasonically cleaned at one time. Sharp instruments must be well-secured; bouncing around in the cleaner dulls them. The contaminated ultrasonic cleaning solution must be changed at the end of each workday, more often if it appears soiled. Then, the basket or cassette and tank must be rinsed, disinfected with a manufacturer-recommended cleaner, rinsed again, and dried.[95,117] Once a month, ultrasonic cleaners should be tested for uniform energy delivery.

Manual precleaning. When instruments must be manually precleaned, health care workers should submerge them in <u>hot</u> soapy water (instead of cold water used for presoaking) and scrub them using a long-handled, stiff-bristled brush. The brush should be sterilized after use.

Packaging Instruments (Step 3)

Table 18 describes procedures for packaging instruments.[95,107,119] All critical and semicritical instruments not scheduled for immediate use should be packaged before sterilization;[100] packaging is possible with all sterilants described in Table 15, except glutaraldehydes and peracetic acid.

Table 18. Instrument Packaging Procedures

1. Use only packaging—pouches, bags, and wrapping materials—recommended by the sterilizer manufacturer. (Appropriate packaging allows the sterilizing agent to penetrate to instruments and does not release unwanted chemicals or nonfast dyes into the sterilizer chamber.)

2. Unclamp locking tools (e.g., needle holders and hemostats), and open hinged instruments (e.g., forceps) so the sterilizing agent can reach all surfaces.

3. Place cleaned and dried instruments in: (a) pouches or bags, or (b) perforated cassettes or trays, which must then be placed in pouches or wrapped, using no more than two layers of wrapping.

4. Use monitoring devices (i.e., chemical indicators and endospore strips), as described in Monitoring Sterilization (Step 5).

5. Press air out of each pouch or bag.

6. Completely seal each package or wrapped item, using autoclave tape or heat-sealing/self-sealing material. Do not use devices (e.g., pins, staples, paper clips) that might puncture the material.

7. Record the date and sterilization cycle number on autoclave tape and attach it to packaging or wrapping, so items can be easily identified if biological monitoring indicates sterilization failure.

Loading Sterilizers (Step 4)

Stacking instrument-containing packages, trays, and cassettes in a sterilizer's chamber, or overloading a chamber, jeopardizes the sterilization process (the sterilizing agent may not reach all parts of the instruments). When a sterilizer lacks racks that separate items, packages and cassettes should be placed on edge and at least a half-inch apart in the chamber.[117]

Autoclave loading tips. Health care workers should:

1. Place empty basins and large trays of instruments at the bottom of the autoclave chamber to prevent condensate from dripping.[108]

2. Line all trays or baskets with a lint-free surgical towel before the packages are loaded (unless manufacturer's instructions state otherwise), to aid absorption of condensate.[119]

Monitoring Sterilization (Step 5)

A proper sterilization cycle, which should be completed without interruption, has two periods:

1. <u>Heat-up</u>—the time it takes for the entire load to reach the selected sterilizing temperature; this varies with load size and composition. (Exceptions are unheated ethylene oxide units and room temperature glutaraldehydes and hydrogen peroxide.) [119]

2. <u>Exposure</u>—the total time required to sterilize the load, with a built-in safety factor for maximum protection.[117]

Although defective temperature and timing gauges and poor-fitting gaskets can cause sterilization cycles to fail, studies have revealed that most failures are the result of human errors, especially overloading chambers, interrupting the cycle, and setting insufficient preheating and exposure times and temperatures.[101][104] To ensure that instruments and equipment are truly sterilized, cycles should be monitored biologically, chemically, and physically. Health care workers must also document and file all relevant data, including:

1. Date and number of cycle.
2. Type of sterilizer.
3. Timing and temperature of cycle.
4. Types and contents of packages containing endospores and chemical indicators.
5. Sterilizer operator's name.
6. Cycle monitoring results.[95]

Biological monitoring. This is the only type of monitoring which indicates whether sterilization has actually occurred; it involves:

1. Processing bacterial endospores through a normal sterilization cycle.[120] The endospores are attached to strips or disks packaged in protective pouches or in vials which also contain ampules of growth medium. Health care workers should follow sterilizer

manufacturers' recommendations for the specific endospore species (either *Bacillus stearothermophilus* or *Bacillus subtilis* variety *niger)* to be used. Recommendations usually include:

a. Processing endospores in the heaviest load to be sterilized during the testing period.

b. Placing a spore strip or disk in one of each type of package (pouch, bag, or cassette) when loads are packaged.

c. Placing spore strips or disks where the least killing power exists (e.g., in the center of the load in steam autoclave, chemical vapor, and static-air dry heat ovens; in the spot farthest from the chamber air inlet in forced-air dry heat units; and in the back of the bottom shelf in a hydrogen peroxide sterilizer).[120]

2. Culturing processed endospores in a steam incubator *(see Fig. 9)* to determine if they were killed. Preferably, incubation should be done in-house; this allows more timely identification of sterilization problems than sending endospores to a sterilization monitoring service, which can take 2 to 7 days to provide confirmation.[95,107]

3. Recalling processed items. When incubated endospores prove viable—an indication that a sterilizing cycle has failed—health care facilities must have an efficient method of recalling items processed since the last acceptable test.[121]

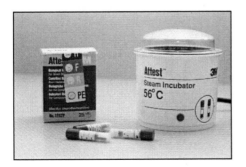

Fig. 9. Biological Monitoring
After being processed through a sterilization cycle, vials containing bacterial endospores and growth medium are incubated. If incubation produces viable spores, instruments processed with them in the sterilizer should be considered contaminated.

The CDC recommends that biological monitoring be done at least weekly;[100] the Department of Veterans Affairs recommends that steam and dry heat sterilizers be biologically monitored daily, and ethylene oxide sterilizers be tested during each cycle.[104] Several states, including Florida, Indiana, Ohio, Oregon, and Washington, mandate endospore testing of dental clinic sterilizers.[107] Biological monitoring should also be done during initial use of a new or repaired sterilizer or a new type of packaging. Implantable devices <u>must</u> be biologically monitored during sterilization, and cannot be used until test results are known.[95]

Glutaraldehyde procedures. When using these liquid sterilants, health care workers should:

1. Place glutaraldehyde in a cleaned, rinsed, and dried decontamination container.

2. Place meticulously precleaned, rinsed, and dried instruments and devices in a perforated tray.

3. Submerge the tray in the chemical and cover the container. (When processing tubing, avoid trapping air bubbles in it and make sure the glutaraldehyde fills it completely.)

Because glutaraldehydes cannot be biologically monitored, health care workers must routinely test solutions to ensure effective concentrations. Testing frequency correlates with use (e.g., if an agent is used daily, it should be tested daily).[96] Even with good test results, manufacturer-specified reuse expiration dates must be adhered to; when test results are poor, the agents must be discarded, even before the expiration dates.

Chemical monitoring. This type of monitoring does not verify sterilization but can indicate whether sterilizers are functioning properly. Integrators—special indicators which change color slowly in response to a sterilizer chamber's temperature—give good results.[95] When placed inside packages or in the center of a load of unwrapped instruments, integrators verify that instruments and devices have been exposed to the desired temperatures.[107,121] However, health care workers should consult manufacturers' instructions on which type of heat-sensitive device works best in specific sterilizers. Ink on these devices should not come into contact with instruments; this could give a false positive, indicating a sterilizer is functioning properly when it is not.[117]

Physical monitoring. Sterilizers' gauges and displays can indicate problems with equipment operation. If sterilizers lack automatic recording devices, health care workers should carefully record readings for temperature, timing, and pressure (in autoclaves) during the cycle, and check them against manufacturers' recommended readings.[95] For vacuum displacement autoclaves, health care workers can use the Bowie-Dick test to check for residual air in the chamber, which can adversely affect steam penetration of items being sterilized.[121]

Handling and Storing Sterilized Instruments (Step 6)

Packaged instruments. Autoclaved instrument packages should be processed through the drying cycle before being removed from the unit, because handling wet paper packages can tear the paper, which allows pathogens to pass through.[95,117]

The dry, sealed packages of sterilized items should be stored in areas which are: (1) clearly designated for "Sterile Items Only"; (2) dry, cool, and well-ventilated; (3) free of dust and heavy traffic; and (4) at least a few inches away from floors, walls, and ceilings. Packages stored for long periods should be sealed inside plastic dust-cover pouches, and checked routinely for possible contamination.[95,117] Shelf life of sterilized instruments relates primarily to whether they become contaminated while stored, not to a particular expiration date.[122,123] Health care workers should check all packages for tears, punctures, or water damage just before opening them.

Unpackaged instruments. Because these instruments are vulnerable to contamination, they must be used immediately after sterilization or stored in a sterile container.[92] In either case, health care workers should don sterile gloves before removing loose instruments <u>one by one, to avoid a sharps injury,</u> from the sterilizer.

To prevent patient exposure to glutaraldehyde, health care workers must don sterile gloves and rinse the processed items thoroughly with sterile water, then dry the items with sterile towels. The term "sterile water" refers to bottled sterile water, which is usually prohibitively expensive, or tap water processed through a 0.1- or 0.2-

micrometer bacterial filter. (Even though filtered water may contain some pathogens less than 0.1 micrometer in size which pass through the filter, it is an improvement over unfiltered tap water which may contain, e.g., *Legionella pneumophila* and *Pseudomonas aeruginosa.*)[124] *(See also Chapter 7, Special Disinfecting Procedures, Endoscopes.)*

Dental handpiece lubrication. For dental handpieces needing lubrication (unless manufacturers' instructions state otherwise), health care workers should:

1. Open sterilizing packaging.

2. Using a spray dispenser reserved for sterilized items, spray water-based lubricant into the handpiece air drive tube.

3. Flush water/air lines and attach the handpiece to the hose.

4. With bur in chuck, blow excess lubricant into the sterile handpiece head cover or onto gauze.[107]

Sterilizer Cleaning

After each use of a sterilizer, the chamber and any racks it contains should be cleaned, following the manufacturer's instructions.

Chain of Events in Clinical Settings

Health care workers must know their roles in the infection control chain of events. In small clinical practices, one person may handle, clean, sterilize or disinfect, and store instruments and devices. In larger facilities, these tasks are assigned to different departments; in these cases, workers should know what the previous department did and not just assume that all prior tasks were performed adequately.

Chapter Summary

1. Sterilization, when done correctly, destroys all forms of microbes.

2. Health care workers must be familiar with: (a) manufacturers' instructions for using all sterilization products; (b) individual hospital and clinical practice policies; and (c) applicable local, state, and federal regulations.

3. Medical instruments classified as <u>critical</u> and most instruments classified as <u>semicritical</u> must be sterilized after each patient.

4. Dry heat sterilization can be biologically monitored, penetrates closed containers, and is noncorrosive for predried items.

5. Ethylene oxide can leave a noxious gas residue on insufficiently aerated rubber and plastic items.

6. Steam autoclaving is the most efficient heat sterilization method; however, autoclaved instrument packages should be processed through the unit's drying cycle before removal.

7. Chemical vapor sterilizers must be carefully monitored for alcohol and ketone levels.

8. "Flash" sterilization should be used only in emergency situations.

9. The six steps in the sterilization process are:

    • Presoaking instruments.

    • Precleaning instruments.

    • Packaging instruments.

    • Loading sterilizers.

    • Monitoring sterilizers.

    • Handling and storing sterilized instruments.

10. For sterilization to be effective, instruments <u>must</u> first be efficiently precleaned.

11. <u>Only biological monitoring</u> indicates whether sterilization has taken place; chemical and physical monitoring indicate only whether a sterilizer is functioning properly.

12. Patients' exposure to glutaraldehyde can be prevented by thoroughly rinsing glutaraldehyde-sterilized items with sterile water, then drying them with sterile towels.

Chapter 7   Disinfection

Disinfection, like sterilization, requires detailed knowledge of manufacturers' instructions, health care facilities' policies, and any applicable laws. This chapter reviews the characteristics, pathogen-killing abilities, and appropriate uses of high-level, intermediate-level, and low-level disinfectants, as well as Occupational Safety and Health Administration (OSHA) requirements and Centers for Disease Control and Prevention (CDC) and Association for Professionals in Infection Control and Epidemiology (APIC) guidelines.

Health care workers performing disinfecting procedures must wear utility gloves and other personal protective equipment as shields from chemicals and infectious substances. Contaminated instruments and devices should be transported from the point of use to the decontamination area in rigid, closed containers. Because organic materials can absorb and inactivate disinfectants, meticulous cleaning and rinsing of instruments and devices are essential first steps. Then, product manufacturers' directions on chemical concentrations and exposure times should be followed.

High-Level Disinfection

This type of disinfection can be used on semicritical-class instruments or devices that cannot tolerate the high temperatures or long exposures to liquid sterilants required for sterilization. Such items include anesthesia breathing circuits, cryosurgical probes, endotracheal tubes, respiratory therapy equipment, and sonographic vaginal probes (which require disinfection even when a condom was used).[96,100] *(See also Special Disinfecting Procedures, Endoscopes.)*

Glutaraldehyde or hydrogen peroxide *(see Table 15)*, or a 1:50 dilution of sodium hypochlorite *(see Table 19)* can be used for high-level disinfection, provided they are compatible with the items being processed. However, only when instruments and devices are rigorously precleaned and exposed to the agents for sufficient time will all microorganisms (except for large numbers of bacterial endospores) be destroyed.[96] Manufacturer-recommended instrument exposure times appear on product labels, but health care workers must also consult with their Infection Control Managers about the high-level disinfection procedures used in their particular facilities.

Table 19. Sodium Hypochlorite High-level disinfection exposure time = 20 minutes or longer.	
Dilution Required to Kill Mycobacteria	**Disadvantages**
1:50 dilution of sodium hypochlorite, providing about 1,000 parts per million available chlorine when product is used within 24 hours of preparation. *(Some hospitals use chloramine-T, which retains chlorine longer than bleach does.)*	This agent can: • Irritate skin and eyes. • Corrode aluminum. • Damage fabric, plastic, and rubber. • Be inactivated by organic matter. • Become ineffective as chlorine is lost.

Intermediate- and Low-Level Disinfection

Intermediate-level disinfection. Although high-level disinfectants can be used as intermediate-level disinfectants, health care facilities often choose iodophors and phenolics for this purpose. These two agents destroy vegetative bacteria, mycobacteria, and most viruses and fungi, but are not sporicidal in manufacturers' recommended dilutions.[96,100,102] They require daily preparation, following product label directions; Table 20 shows other characteristics to be considered. Hydrotherapy tanks, although classified as semicritical, can be disinfected at the intermediate level.[96]

Table 20. Iodophors and Phenolics **Intermediate-level disinfection exposure time = 10 minutes or longer.**[†]	
Agents:[††]	**Disadvantages**

Iodophor germicidal detergent solutions.	1. Iodophors can:
	  • Corrode metal and stain light-colored vinyl.
	  • Be inactivated by organic matter (rigorous precleaning is required).
	  • Become ineffective as iodine is lost.
	2. Iodophors do not destroy bacterial endospores.

Phenolic germicidal detergent solutions.	1. Phenolics can:
	  • Irritate tissues exposed to them.
	  • Degrade soft plastic and etch glass.
	  • Be inactivated by soaps.
	  • Cause hyperbilirubinemia in infants whose incubators or bassinets are cleaned with them (e.g., following manufacturer's recommendations; some are suitable if wiped off after waiting for prescribed time. Equipment should not be in use at the time).
	2. Phenolics do not destroy bacterial endospores.

[†] Consult manufacturers' recommendations.

[††] Products must be Environmental Protection Agency (EPA)-registered as hospital disinfectants, labeled with the appropriate EPA number, tuberculocidal, and virucidal for at least lipophilic and hydrophilic viruses (see Chapter 6, Susceptibility of Microbes).

Low-level disinfection. This type of disinfection kills some viruses and fungi and most bacteria, but not mycobacteria and endospores. Low-level disinfection is used for noncritical-class devices (i.e., those which contact intact skin but <u>not</u> mucous membranes), including bedpans, blood pressure cuffs, crutches, electrocardiographic leads, splints, stethoscopes, and x-ray heads and shields.

Health care workers should check with their Infection Control Managers regarding choices of low-level disinfectants and their uses. Intermediate-level disinfectants can, of course, be used for noncritical-class devices, but, for items not contaminated with potentially infectious substances (e.g., blood, saliva, mucus, and feces), many health care facilities choose a 1:500 dilution of sodium hypochlorite. Some facilities allow use of 70% to 90% alcohols for wiping off thermometers, stethoscopes, and rubber stoppers of multiple-dose medication vials.[96]

Clinical surfaces. Health care workers should consider all clinical and hospital room surfaces to be potentially contaminated, and routinely disinfect them, unless protective coverings *(see below)* are used. Table 21 shows OSHA housekeeping requirements.[23]

Table 21. Housekeeping and OSHA Compliance	
Persons	**Responsibilities**
Employers' requirements.	1. Write and implement an appropriate schedule for disinfection, based on the types of surfaces, soils, and tasks or procedures performed in the specific workplace areas to be cleaned. 2. Ensure that the workplace is maintained in a clean and sanitary condition.

Health care workers' requirements.	1. Clean and disinfect all environmental or work surfaces which have had any contact with blood or other potentially infectious materials, using the "spray-wipe-spray" method:
	   a. Spray environmental and work surfaces with a <u>cleaning agent</u>.
	   b. Wipe the surfaces vigorously with paper towels; if this does not remove all visible contamination, scrub surfaces with a brush.
	   c. Spray surfaces with your health care facility's choice of <u>disinfectant</u>; allow the surface to remain wet for at least 10 minutes, <u>or,</u> if you do not use a spray container to apply liquids (e.g., to avoid shorting electrical switches), saturate paper towels with liquids just before applying them to the surfaces.
	   d. To avoid transferring disinfectant to patients' skin or clothing, wipe the surface dry after 10 or more minutes.[100,107]
	 2. Inspect, on a regularly scheduled basis, all reusable bins, pails, cans, and similar receptacles which are reasonably likely to become contaminated with blood or other potentially infectious materials. Clean and intermediate-level disinfect these receptacles when they are visibly contaminated.

For disinfection to be effective, surfaces must be meticulously precleaned *(see Table 21, steps 1a and 1b).* Surfaces should be disinfected after:

1. Treating a patient or completing any task in a clinical laboratory.

2. An event involving overt contamination or any spill of blood or other potentially infectious materials (disinfect <u>immediately</u>).

3. The work shift ends, if the surface was contaminated after its last cleaning.[96]

Environmental Protection Agency (EPA)-registered disinfectants labeled as effective against human immunodeficiency virus (HIV) and hepatitis B virus can be used to disinfect blood-contaminated environmental surfaces, <u>provided such surfaces have not become contaminated with agents, or volumes/concentrations of agents, for which higher-level disinfection is recommended.</u> Effectiveness of disinfection is governed by strict adherence to label instructions. Some product labels state that all blood must be cleaned thoroughly before applying the disinfectant and stipulate the amount of time that the surface must be left wet with the disinfectant to kill the HIV or hepatitis B virus.

Protective Coverings

Appropriate covers on disinfected clinical surfaces and noncritical-class devices serve as barriers to contamination. *(See Figs. 10 and 11.)* All covers must be impervious to fluids and thick enough to resist puncturing by the surfaces or devices they are protecting. Some plastic coverings are sold in shapes that fit specific items.[95]

OSHA-required use of protective coverings involves:

1. Replacing plastic wrap, aluminum foil, or imperviously backed absorbent paper, used to cover equipment and environmental surfaces, when the coverings become overtly contaminated.

2. Removing and replacing such protective coverings at the end of the work shift, if any procedure might have contaminated the coverings during the shift. (The CDC recommends that, in dental settings, health care workers replace coverings after treating each patient.)[100]

When replacing coverings that are visibly, or even possibly, contaminated, health care workers should: (1) discard the removed covers as regulated waste, discussed in Chapter 8; (2) remove their gloves; (3) wash their hands; (4) reglove; and (5) re-cover the surfaces and devices. <u>However</u>, if contamination occurs during removal of a covering, the original disinfection process must be repeated.[100]

Disposable protective coverings are suitable for use on clinical surfaces and noncritical-class items such as:

1. Furniture (e.g., counters, stools, and chairs).

2. Containers, hoses, and trays, and hardware (e.g., handles, knobs, buttons, and switches).

3. X-ray equipment (e.g., extension cone, tube head, swivel arms, and daylight loader interior).

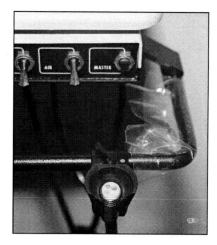 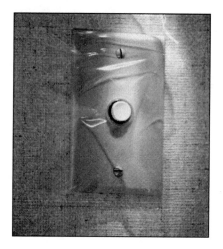

Fig. 10. Disposable Plastic Surface Barriers
Coverings protect a dental unit handle (left) and an x-ray exposure button (right).

Special Disinfecting Procedures

The choice of agents to be used for disinfecting endoscopes, dental unit waterlines, and various dental materials varies with health care facilities.

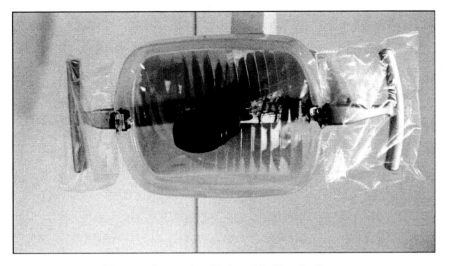

Fig. 11. Operating Light with Plastic Cover

Endoscope Disinfection

There have been about 400 reported cases of infection following either gastrointestinal endoscopy or bronchoscopy; patients' clinical responses ranged from asymptomatic pathogen colonization to death.[96] Health care workers should consult the APIC guidelines for specific details of high-level disinfection of flexible endoscopes (semicritical-class instruments), which cannot be sterilized using heat or ethylene oxide.[110] Basic procedures are:

1. Meticulously clean the internal channels, ports, and external surfaces with an enzymatic detergent and water.

2. Rinse and drain the channels.

3. Immerse the endoscope in high-level disinfectant, and perfuse the agent into the channels (i.e., air, water, and suction/biopsy).

4. Keep the endoscope immersed for a minimum of 20 minutes. When endoscopes have been thoroughly precleaned using the standard process and need to be reused quickly, some facilities use the APIC 20/20 glutaraldehyde guidelines: expose the instruments for 20 minutes at 68°F (20°C), instead of the 45- to 90-minute

exposure at up to 77°F (25°C) that appears on manufacturers' labels.[124]

5. Rinse the endoscope, internally and externally, three times with sterile water, <u>or,</u> if this is not possible, rinse once with tap water, then rinse and flush internally with 70% to 90% alcohol.

6. Don sterile gloves, dry the endoscope with forced air, and store it in a way that prevents recontamination.[96]

Dental Unit Water Line Disinfection

According to the general recommendations of the CDC, dental offices should:[9]

1. Use water that meets Environmental Protection Agency regulatory standards for drinking water (i.e., 500 or fewer colony-forming units [CFUs] per milliliter of heterotrophic water bacteria) for routine dental treatment output water.

2. Consult with the dental unit manufacturer for appropriate methods and equipment to maintain the recommended quality of dental water.

3. Follow recommendations for monitoring water quality provided by the manufacturer of the unit or water line treatment product.

4. Discharge water and air for a minimum of 20 to 30 seconds after each patient, from any device connected to the dental water system that enters the patient's mouth (e.g., handpieces, ultrasonic scalers, air/water syringes).

5. Consult with the dental unit manufacturer on the need for periodic maintenance of antiretraction mechanisms.

Boil water advisory. When a boil water advisory is in effect, water from the public water system should not be delivered to the patient through any dental equipment that uses the public water system (e.g., dental operative unit, ultrasonic scaler), nor should water from the public water system be used for dental treatment, patient rinsing, or handwashing. Alcohol-based hand rubs that do not require water should be used for handwashing. When the advisory is lifted, flush dental water lines and faucets for 1 to 5 minutes before using for patient care. Check with the local water utility for any specific guidance on flushing of water lines. Disinfect dental water lines as recommended by the dental unit manufacturer.[9]

Dental Material Disinfection

Before shipping items which have had patient contact to a dental laboratory, health care workers should: (1) remove any blood and saliva from them; (2) disinfect the items and their containers; and (3) label all these as disinfected. The ADA recommends that health care workers carefully follow manufacturers' instructions for disinfecting impressions because material-disinfectant compatibilities vary greatly.[92] Other items should receive at least the following high- or intermediate-level disinfection:

1. Wax bites or rims—disinfect with iodophors, using the spray-wipe-spray method.

2. Fixed prostheses (metal or porcelain)—immerse in glutaraldehyde for 20 or more minutes.

3. Removable partials (metal or acrylic) and removable dentures (acrylic or porcelain)—immerse in iodophors for 10 or more minutes.

4. Stone casts—spray-wipe-spray or immerse in iodophors for 10 or more minutes or sodium hypochlorite for 20 minutes or longer.[92,100]

When incoming prostheses and other items are not labeled as disinfected, laboratory health care workers should: (1) dispose of packing materials as regulated waste; (2) disinfect the items (as indicated above) and their containers; and (3) disinfect items and containers again, prior to returning them to the dental clinic. If incoming items and their containers are not labeled as disinfected, clinical health care workers must disinfect them. The disinfectant must be thoroughly rinsed from each item before it is placed into a patient's mouth.[92]

Within clinical facilities, laboratory health care workers should disinfect dental lathe units twice a day, and reusable brushes and stones at least daily. (Rag wheels must be washed and autoclaved after use for each case.) For each item, health care workers should dispense only a small quantity of pumice in a disposable container, then discard excess pumice and the container.[95] Pumice can be mixed with 5 parts sodium hypochlorite to 100 parts distilled water; adding 3 parts green soap to the solution keeps pumice suspended.[92,117]

Dental Radiographic Equipment

Gloves should be worn when taking radiographs and handling contaminated film packets. Other PPE (e.g., protective eyewear, mask, gown) should be used when spattering of patient body fluids is likely. Whenever possible, only heat-tolerant or disposable intraoral x-ray accessories (e.g., film holders, positioning devices) should be used; heat-tolerant devices should be cleaned and heat sterilized between patients. Exposed radiographs must be transported and handled aseptically to prevent contamination of development equipment. Heat-sensitive semicritical devices (e.g., intraoral cameras, electronic periodontal probes) that cannot be heat sterilized should undergo high-level disinfection according to the manufacturer's directions.

Digital radiographic sensors should be cleaned and heat sterilized, or undergo high-level disinfection, between patients. If the equipment cannot tolerate these procedures, then they should be protected with an FDA-cleared barrier to reduce gross contamination. Consult with the manufacturer for methods of sterilization and disinfection of digital radiographic sensors.[9]

Chapter Summary

1. Disinfectants are categorized as high-level, intermediate-level, and low-level, and have differing characteristics, pathogen-killing abilities, and uses.

2. The same agents are used for high-level disinfection as for room-temperature sterilization, but instrument exposure times are much shorter during disinfection.

3. Although sodium hypochlorite (1:50 dilution) is an effective high-level disinfectant, it has a number of negative qualities.

4. Iodophors and phenolics are acceptable intermediate-level disinfectants that inactivate mycobacteria, vegetative bacteria, and most viruses and fungi.

5. All clinical and hospital room surfaces should be treated as potentially contaminated, and routinely precleaned and disinfected.

6. The "spray-wipe-spray" method should be used to clean and disinfect environmental and work surfaces.

7. Disposable protective coverings are suitable for use on certain surfaces and noncritical-class items.

8. APIC guidelines provide specific details of high-level disinfection of flexible endoscopes.

9. Health care workers should discharge water and air for a minimum of 20 to 30 seconds after each dental patient, from any device connected to the dental unit water system that entered the patient's mouth.

10. Health care workers should carefully follow manufacturers' instructions for disinfecting dental impressions because material-disinfectant compatibilities vary greatly.

11. Exposed dental radiographs must be transported and handled aseptically to prevent contamination of development equipment.

Chapter 8   Hazard Controls

The Occupational Safety and Health Administration (OSHA) requires health care workers to perform all procedures involving blood or other potentially infectious materials in a manner that minimizes splashing, spraying, spattering, and droplet generation. Reducing the likelihood of occupational exposure involves use of:

1. Work-practice controls that alter the way in which tasks are performed (e.g., always activate safety features).

2. Engineering controls that isolate or remove bloodborne pathogens from the workplace (e.g., use of sharps-only waste containers). OSHA requires that employers regularly examine and maintain, or replace, engineering controls to ensure their effectiveness.[23]

Sharps: Handle with Care!

OSHA defines contaminated sharps as any contaminated objects that can penetrate the skin, including, but not limited to, needles, scalpel blades, curettes, dental burs, and extracted teeth. Health care workers should check their states' regulations for any modifications to this definition. Table 22 shows OSHA-required procedures for sharps use and disposal of them when they are contaminated.[23] For tips on sharpening, using, and discarding sharps, follow the table.

Table 22. Sharps and OSHA Compliance	
Persons	**Responsibilities**
Employers' requirements.	1. Ensure that contaminated needles are not recapped or removed unless no feasible alternative can be demonstrated or such action is required by a specific medical procedure. (Such recapping or needle removal must be accomplished using a mechanical device or a one-handed scoop technique.)
	2. Prohibit employees from shearing or breaking contaminated needles.
	3. Ensure that containers for contaminated sharps are: a. Easily accessible to employees and located close to the immediate area where sharps are used or usually found. b. Maintained upright throughout use. c. Replaced routinely to prevent overfill. d. Puncture-resistant and meet requirements 1a through 1c in Table 23.
	4. Ensure that contaminated, reusable sharps are stored or processed so that employees need not put their hands into containers holding these sharps.
	5. Provide effective sharps safety devices, after receiving input from nonmanagerial, frontline employees who have been involved in the identification, evaluation, and selection of such devices* (e.g., syringes with retractable needles or a protective shield; blunt-tip blood-drawing needles; and needleless or protected-needle intravenous systems).**
Employees' requirements.	1. Discard contaminated sharps immediately in containers described above.
	2. When reusable sharps containers are used (seldom), avoid opening or emptying them manually or in any manner that could cause a percutaneous injury. Clean and disinfect only <u>empty</u> sharps containers.
	3. Avoid picking up potentially contaminated broken glassware by hand; such glassware must be cleaned up using mechanical means (i.e., a brush and dust pan, tongs, or forceps).

* Added to section 1910.1030(c)(1) of OSHA's "Occupational Exposure to Bloodborne Pathogens; Final Rule." For details, see "Needlesticks and Other Sharps Injuries; Final Rule," *Federal Register,* 66(12):5318-5325, January 18, 2001.[125]

** See *NIOSH Alert: Preventing Needlestick Injuries in Health Care Settings,* National Institute for Occupational Safety and Health (NIOSH), November 1999.[126] www.cdc.gov/niosh

Tips on Sharps in General

1. Avoid unnecessary use of needles and other sharps.

2. Keep the sharp end of handheld instruments angled away from yourself, coworkers, and patients. Fig. 12 illustrates the <u>incorrect</u> procedure, using a needle as an example.

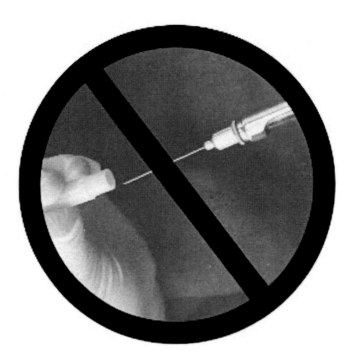

Fig. 12. Don't Do This!
Never aim a needle at yourself or use two hands to recap a needle.

3. Use forceps, a suture holder, or other instrument for suturing. Do not hold tissue with your fingers when suturing or cutting.

4. Use a one-handed technique if organic debris must be cleaned from an instrument tip during patient treatment (e.g., swipe the tip across gauze taped to the instrument tray).[23,92,102]

5. Do not leave sharps on a procedure field.

6. Pass sharp instruments by use of designated "safe zones."

7. Never pick up a handful of sharp instruments; pick up each one individually, using forceps.

8. Disassemble sharp equipment by use of forceps or other devices.

9. Dispose of a scalpel blade by clamping a hemostat on the retentive end of the blade, then removing the blade and depositing it in a sharps container.

10. Make sure instruments are sterilized before sharpening them, and use single-use, sterile sharpening stones, or ultrasonically cleaned and heat-sterilized stones.

Tips on Use and Disposal of Needles

1. Use needles with safety devices *(see Table 22, item 5)*. During NIOSH's 4-year study of nearly 5,000 percutaneous injuries in hospitals, hypodermic needles were associated with 29% and winged-steel (butterfly-type) needles with 13% of the injuries.[126]

2. Do not walk any distance holding an uncapped needle.

3. Use disposable needles whenever possible, to avoid the risks involved in sterilizing nondisposable needles. In some cases, disposable needles are mandatory (e.g., in Florida, for acupuncturists). Health care workers should know their states' laws on this subject.

4. Discard single-use, disposable syringes and needles (uncapped); never attempt to sterilize them.

5. Discard used needles, <u>immediately after use</u>, in a puncture-resistant container. Do not allow uncovered used needles to remain on an instrument tray.

6. Do not recap, bend, or break needles before discarding them in the sharps container; <u>never touch a used needle</u>. When needle recapping is necessary during treatments involving multiple injections from a single syringe, use a one-handed technique *(see Figs. 13 and 14),* <u>not</u> the two-handed technique shown in Fig. 12.

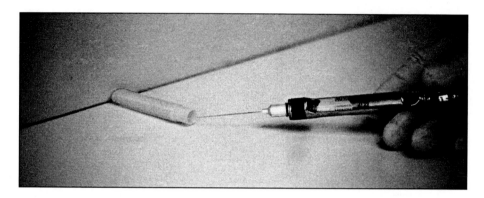

Fig. 13. The Scoop Technique

After using one hand and the scoop technique to recap a needle, you should tighten the cap by grasping it at its base (near its orifice). Do not grasp the top end of the cap, because the needle might pierce it during the cap-tightening process. Recapping is done when multiple injections from a syringe are needed during a patient's treatment.

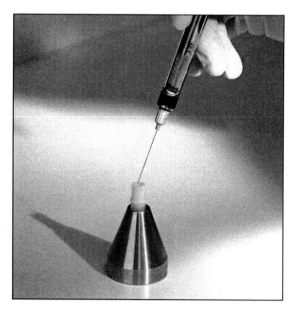

Fig. 14. Needle Recapping Stand

Use one hand to place the needle into the cap, which sits in the weighted stand. Do not touch the stand with your other hand during the recapping process.

Regulated Waste

OSHA defines regulated waste as:

1. Liquid or semi-liquid blood or other potentially infectious materials *(defined in Chapter 1, Algorithm 1 footnote).*

2. Contaminated items that, if compressed, would release blood or other potentially infectious materials in a liquid or semi-liquid state.

3. Items caked with dried blood or other potentially infectious materials and capable of releasing these materials.

4. Contaminated sharps.

5. Pathological and microbiological wastes containing blood or other potentially infectious materials.[23]

Proper containment, labeling, and disposal of regulated waste (also known as biomedical, biohazardous, or infectious waste) require strict engineering controls. Table 23 shows OSHA requirements.[23]

Table 23. Regulated Waste and OSHA Compliance
Employers and health care workers must ensure that:

1. Regulated waste is placed in containers that are:
  a. Constructed to secure all contents and prevent leakage of fluids during handling, storage, transport, or shipping.
  b. Closable <u>and closed prior to removal</u>, to prevent spillage or protrusion of the contents during handling, storage, transport, or shipping.
  c. Labeled or color-coded *(see Table 24).*

2. Containers that become contaminated on the outside are placed in second containers that fulfill requirements 1a through 1c.
3. Nonpuncture-resistant containers holding waste able to puncture them are placed in second containers that are puncture-resistant and fulfill requirements 1a through 1c.

State and local laws often impose additional directives on regulated waste generators; for example: (1) permits; and (2) detailed, written waste management plans. When permitted by laws and clinic or hospital policies, patient-care items <u>not</u> fitting OSHA's definition of regulated waste can be discarded with ordinary trash.

Containers

Each clinical operatory should have both a sharps-only container *(right)* and a regulated waste container that meet OSHA requirements *(see Tables 22 and 23)*. Both must have a highly visible biohazard warning label affixed to them *(for exceptions, see Table 24)*. The waste container should be lined with a thick plastic "red bag" (check local and state requirements).[127] Health care workers should <u>not</u> mix ordinary trash with regulated wastes.

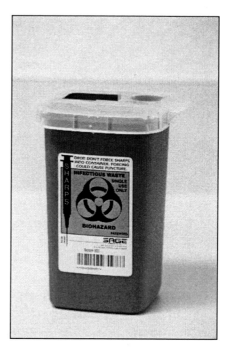

Fig. 15. Sharps Container

Warning and Identification Labels

Table 24 describes OSHA warning label requirements, as well as exceptions to them.[23] Health care workers should check local and state laws for specifics on use of the label (e.g., Florida law requires that, on sharps containers, "red bags," and outer containers, the biohazard <u>symbol</u> be at least 1 inch in diameter on items measuring less than 19 by 14 inches and at least 6 inches in diameter on those measuring 19 by 14 inches or more).[127]

All containers should be labeled with the waste generator's name and address, as well as information that identifies contracted waste haulers, if used *(see Disposal of Regulated Waste, item 1)*.

Table 24. Biohazard Warning Labels and OSHA Compliance
Requirements for employers and health care workers: 1. Ensure that warning labels include the biohazard symbol and the word BIOHAZARD *(see Fig. 15)*. 2. Ensure that warning labels are fluorescent orange or orange-red, or predominantly so, with the lettering or biohazard symbol in a contrasting color. 3. Ensure that warning labels are affixed to: (a) regulated-waste containers, refrigerators, and freezers containing blood or other potentially infectious materials; and (b) other containers used to store, transport, or ship such materials. Labels should be affixed by string, wire, adhesive, or any other means that will prevent their loss or unintentional removal. 4. Ensure that warning labels are affixed to contaminated equipment, and that the labels state which parts of the equipment are contaminated.
Exceptions: 1. Red bags or red containers may be used without labels (<u>unless</u> state or local laws mandate otherwise). 2. Containers of blood or blood components and products released for transfusion or other clinical uses need only bear labels describing their contents. 3. For storage, transport, shipment, or disposal, <u>individual</u> containers of blood or other potentially infectious materials need only be placed in an appropriate, labeled container. 4. Decontaminated regulated waste need not be labeled or color-coded. 5. In facilities using Universal Precautions[†] in the handling of all specimens, specimen containers need not be labeled <u>provided</u> they are recognizable as containing specimens and that such specimens and containers remain within the facility.

[†] OSHA requires use of Universal Precautions, now included in Standard Precautions. *(See Chapter 1.)*

Disposal of Regulated Waste

OSHA requires that disposal of all regulated waste be carried out in accordance with federal, state, county, and territorial regulations. <u>Final responsibility for proper disposal of the waste always lies with the health care facility that generates it.</u>[95]

The following three methods are used, but health care workers must know the laws in their specific states or localities regarding each method:

1. <u>A registered waste hauler.</u> Most health care facilities contract with a registered hauler who transports their regulated waste off-site, treats it, and disposes of it. "Red bags" and sharps containers (or

exterior containers in which these items are placed) must be labeled with the hauler's name, address, registration number, and 24-hour telephone number. The hauler must provide a receipt for each shipment of waste and a subsequent manifest describing the exact treatment and disposal of the waste. Health care facilities should keep both documents for at least 3 years.[127]

2. Waste generator hauling. Some states allow health care facilities to transport less than 25 pounds of their regulated waste in their own transport vehicles to a registered storage or treatment facility.[127]

3. In-house treatment of waste. Some states allow health care facilities to steam autoclave or incinerate regulated waste. Some states also allow compacting of pretreated waste.

Liquid Waste

The CDC states that blood, suctioned fluids, or other liquid waste may be poured carefully into a drain connected to a sanitary sewer system. If this is done, sink traps and evacuation lines should be flushed or purged at least once a day to reduce bacterial growth.[92,100] However, some state and local governments restrict the volume of blood and chemicals allowed in their sewers, and health care workers should check all applicable laws.[95]

Hazardous Chemicals

During certain sterilization and disinfection procedures, health care workers may be exposed to hazardous chemicals; examples include:

1. Glutaraldehydes, ethylene oxide, and unsaturated chemical vapor, all of which require proper ventilation during sterilization procedures (see Table 15, for OSHA-mandated exposure limits).

2. The lead oxide in the white powder residue in boxes used to store dental intraoral radiograph film. Because lead oxide cannot be removed adequately, the CDC has issued an alert recommending that the film packets stored in lead-lined boxes and the boxes themselves be discarded.[128] Films, both exposed and unexposed, are best stored in a room other than where radiographs are exposed.

3. Mercury vapor in dental operatories, associated with the use of amalgam. The American Dental Association recommends that dental professionals use: (1) only precapsulated alloys; (2) an amalgamator with a completely enclosed arm; and (3) high-volume evacuation when removing or finishing amalgam. A dosimeter can be used to monitor the dental operatory air for mercury vapor. The OSHA limit for mercury vapor is 50 micrograms per cubic meter (time-weighted-average) in an 8-hour work shift over a 40-hour workweek.[129]

Hazard Communication Program. OSHA considers a chemical hazardous if it is combustible, explosive, flammable, unstable, water-reactive, carcinogenic, toxic, corrosive, or an irritant or sensitizer. Employers should consult OSHA's "Hazard Communication; Final Rule,"[130] which requires them to provide a written Hazard Communication Program specific to their workplace.

Labels. OSHA also requires chemical manufacturers, importers, and distributors to label shipping and clinical-use containers with:

1. The identity of the chemical—the name that appears on the Material Safety Data Sheet (MSDS) which the manufacturer must send with the initial shipment of the product.
2. Appropriate hazard warnings.
3. The manufacturer's name, address, and telephone number.[130]

Material Safety Data Sheets. These must include:

1. The chemical's name, its hazardous ingredients, and physical or chemical characteristics (e.g., the chemical's reactivity under various conditions).
2. The telephone number to be called in the event of a chemical emergency involving the product, and appropriate emergency first-aid procedures.
3. Signs and symptoms of overexposure to the chemical, and health hazards associated with its use.
4. Control measures (e.g., ventilation and personal protective equipment) required for safe handling and use of the chemical.

Manufacturers who make any changes in their chemical products must supply new Material Safety Data Sheets to customers.[130]

Hazard Reporting

The Occupational Safety and Health Act of 1970 requires that all employers prominently display the poster "Job Safety & Health Protection," which explains employees' rights to file complaints about unsafe working conditions. (Employers in states administering their own OSHA-approved programs must post their states' equivalent posters.)

Employees or their representatives have the right to file complaints with the nearest OSHA office *(see Appendix A)*, requesting an inspection if they believe hazardous conditions exist in their workplaces. OSHA will withhold, on request, the names of employees registering such complaints. The employer will be asked to select an employer representative to accompany the OSHA compliance officer during the inspection. An authorized representative of the employees, if any, also has the right to go along. The compliance officer has the right to consult with a "reasonable number" of employees.[131]

If the OSHA compliance officer believes an employer has violated the Act, he or she issues a citation stating the time period within which the alleged violation must be corrected. The citation must be prominently displayed at or near the place of the alleged violation for a minimum of 3 days, or until the condition is corrected, <u>whichever is longer.</u>

Chapter Summary

1. Use of work-practice controls and engineering controls can reduce health care workers' likelihood of occupational exposure to infectious substances.

2. OSHA requires employers to provide effective sharps safety devices, after receiving input from nonmanagerial, frontline employees.

3. Contaminated sharps must be discarded immediately in containers that meet OSHA specifications.

4.   OSHA requires that all items contaminated with blood or other potentially infectious materials be treated as regulated waste.

5.   Regulated waste containers must be red and/or specifically labeled.

6.   In most states, blood, suctioned fluids, or other liquid waste, <u>in specified amounts</u>, may be poured into a drain connected to a sanitary sewer system.

7.   OSHA has set limits for workers' exposure to glutaraldehydes, ethylene oxide, unsaturated chemical vapor, and mercury vapor; areas in which these chemicals are used must have proper ventilation.

8.   Containers of hazardous chemicals must be labeled with the name of the chemical, appropriate hazard warnings, and the manufacturer's name, address, and telephone number.

9.   Employees who believe that hazardous conditions exist in their workplaces have the right to file complaints with the nearest OSHA office.

Chapter 9   Planning and Training

This chapter discusses administrative measures designed to guard against transmission of infectious diseases. These include: (1) the Occupational Safety and Health Administration (OSHA)-required Exposure Control Plan and personnel training; and (2) Centers for Disease Control and Prevention (CDC)-recommended personnel medical evaluations.

Exposure Control Plan

OSHA requires all employers with employees at risk of occupational exposure to bloodborne pathogens to write an Exposure Control Plan; this includes an exposure determination for each employee, as well as the elements listed in Table 25.[23]

Infection Control Manager

The Infection Control Manager for a health care facility supervises and implements the OSHA-required Exposure Control Plan. He or she also makes certain that employees comply with other infection control procedures [e.g., those recommended by the CDC and Association for Professionals in Infection Control and Epidemiology (APIC)].

Table 25. Exposure Control Plan and OSHA Compliance

Requirements for employers:

1. Produce a written Exposure Control Plan designed to eliminate or minimize employees' occupational exposure to bloodborne pathogens.

2. Ensure that the Exposure Control Plan contains <u>at least</u> the following elements:
   a. An exposure determination made without regard to employees' use of personal protective equipment; it must include lists of:
      - All job classifications in which <u>all</u> employees risk occupational exposure.
      - Job classifications in which <u>some</u> employees risk occupational exposure, and tasks and procedures (or groups of closely related tasks and procedures) these employees perform which involve risk of occupational exposure.
   b. The schedule and method of implementing compliance with all requirements of OSHA's "Occupational Exposure to Bloodborne Pathogens; Final Rule."

3. Ensure that a copy of the Exposure Control Plan is accessible to all employees.

4. Review and update the Exposure Control Plan at least annually <u>and</u> whenever necessary to reflect:
   a. New or modified tasks and procedures that affect occupational exposure.
   b. New or changed employee jobs involving occupational exposure.
   c. Technologic changes that eliminate or reduce exposure to bloodborne pathogens. This includes documenting: (1) input solicited from nonmanagerial, frontline employees on effective sharps safety devices *(see Table 22);* and (2) consideration and implementation of appropriate commercially available, effective, safer medical devices.

5. Make the Exposure Control Plan available to the Director of the National Institute for Occupational Safety and Health and the Assistant Secretary of Labor for Occupational Safety and Health (or their designated representatives), upon request, for examination and copying.

Examples of an Infection Control Manager's responsibilities are:

1. Assisting employers to train and educate all new employees, and to retrain employees annually at a minimum *(see Table 26).*

2. Maintaining files of OSHA-required records and documents *(see Chapter 10).*

3. Ensuring that sterilizer biological monitors are processed at least weekly *[Chapter 6, Monitoring Sterilization (Step 5)].*

4. Managing quality control, cost-effectiveness, and inventory.

In outpatient clinical practices, Infection Control Managers oversee readiness of treatment rooms by ensuring that they are: (a) ready for treatment of the first patients each workday; (b) ready to receive subsequent patients; and (c) prepared for closing at the end of the workday.[132] (*See Appendix C for a checklist.*)

Employee Medical Evaluations

New employees must not be given initial assignments which would pose undue risk of infection to themselves, other personnel, patients, or visitors; therefore, the CDC recommends that employers ensure that new employees have on record:

1. <u>Health inventories</u> which include:

    a. Vaccination status, history of vaccine-preventable diseases, and presence of conditions which contraindicate use of vaccines or immune globulins. *(See also Appendix B.)*

    b. History of any conditions that might predispose health care workers to acquire or transmit infectious diseases (e.g., chronic draining infections or open wounds, dermatologic problems, immunosuppressive ailments, or tuberculosis).

    c. Allergies to latex.

2. <u>Physical examinations and laboratory tests</u>. These may be indicated by health inventory data or required by local public health ordinances.[1]

Except when OSHA-required, individual employers can decide whether items 1 and 2 are provided free of charge. OSHA-required employee medical records are described in Chapter 10 (Table 27).

Employee Training

Health care workers at risk of exposure to pathogens or chemicals must be trained to recognize, evaluate, and, when possible, control the hazards. The training must comply with federal, state, and local regulations, and should include, when feasible, specialized training on infection risks associated with specific jobs.

Bloodborne Pathogens

OSHA requires employers to provide free intensive training to employees at the time of initial assignment to (but <u>before</u> they perform) any tasks that might expose them to bloodborne pathogens *(see Table 26).*[23] Bloodborne pathogen training must be provided for new employees (full-time, part-time, and temporary); all of these employees must be retrained at least annually <u>and</u> whenever new occupational exposure risks occur. Contractual workers (e.g., evening janitorial workers) should be given a written maintenance plan, in languages they understand, to help them avoid: (1) occupational exposure; and (2) contaminating the clinic. This information must be provided orally to reading-handicapped persons.[132]

All Contagious Diseases

In addition to OSHA-required employee training about bloodborne pathogens, the CDC recommends that training stress the importance of:

1. Complying with Standard and Transmission-Based Precautions.

2. Participating in vaccination and personnel screening programs.

3. Reporting illnesses (work- and nonwork-related), including these signs or symptoms: (a) jaundice; (b) vesicular, pustular, or weeping skin lesions or rashes; (c) a cough lingering longer than 2 weeks; (d) a temperature over 103°F (39.4°C), lasting longer than 2 days; and (e) prolonged gastrointestinal illness.[1]

Hazardous Chemicals

OSHA requires employers to provide free training to employees <u>before</u> they are exposed to hazardous chemicals <u>and</u> whenever a new hazard is introduced into their work areas. The training must include:

1. The requirements of OSHA's "Hazard Communication; Final Rule."

2. The location and contents of the health care facility's: (a) Hazard Communication Program; and (b) lists of, and Material Safety Data Sheets for, all hazardous chemicals used in the clinic.

3. How to use the information on chemical-container labels and in Material Safety Data Sheets, including what to do in case of exposure.[130]

Table 26. Employee Training and OSHA Compliance

Employers must:

1. Ensure that all employees at risk of occupational exposure to bloodborne pathogens participate in free training programs, provided during working hours:

    a. At the time of their initial assignments to tasks involving occupational exposure.

    b. At least annually thereafter, within 1 year of their previous training.

2. Provide additional training when changes (e.g., modification or institution of tasks or procedures) affect employees' risks of occupational exposure; this training may be limited to explaining how to deal with any new exposures.

3. Ensure that training materials are appropriate in content and vocabulary to the educational level, literacy, and language of employees.

4. Ensure that training programs contain, at a minimum:

    a. An accessible copy of the regulatory text of "OSHA's Occupational Exposure to Bloodborne Pathogens; Final Rule" and an explanation of its contents.

    b. A general explanation of the epidemiology and symptoms of bloodborne diseases.

    c. Explanations of:

    (1) Bloodborne pathogen transmission modes.

    (2) The employer's Exposure Control Plan and how employees can obtain a copy of it.

    (3) Appropriate methods for recognizing tasks and other activities that may involve exposure to blood and other potentially infectious materials.

    (4) Uses and limitations of techniques to prevent or reduce exposure: engineering controls (including sharps safety devices), work practices, and personal protective equipment.

    (5) Procedures to follow if an exposure incident occurs, including the reporting method and postexposure medical follow-up available to exposed employees.

    (6) OSHA-required signs and labels and/or color-coding *(see Table 24).*

    d. Information on:

    (1) Types, basis for selection, proper use, location, removal, handling, decontamination, and disposal of personal protective equipment.

    (2) Appropriate actions to take and persons to contact in an emergency involving blood or other potentially infectious materials.

    (3) Hepatitis B vaccine, including its efficacy, safety, administration method, free-of-charge availability, and the benefits of being vaccinated.

    e. An opportunity for interactive questions and answers with the trainer.

5. Ensure that trainers are knowledgeable about the training programs' subject matter as it relates to the workplace involved.

6. Maintain accurate, continuous records of employee training *(see Chapter 10).*

Training Methods

OSHA requires that qualified employee trainers have comprehensive, up-to-date knowledge about infection control; they must also:

1. Provide training at levels and in languages comprehensible to all trainees.
2. Avoid training solely by means of text, films, videotapes, or generic computer software.[95]

In addition to teaching health care workers how to protect themselves and their patients against infection, the training should prepare health care workers to communicate clearly with patients about basic infection control measures used in their health care facilities. Further information on employee training can be obtained from OSHA *(see Appendix A)*.

Required Documents

Health care facilities must keep the following documents where employees can easily refer to them:

1. OSHA's "Occupational Exposure to Bloodborne Pathogens; Final Rule."
2. The facility's Exposure Control Plan *(see Table 25)*.
3. Up-to-date federal, state, and local laws regulating the facility.
4. OSHA's "Hazard Communication; Final Rule."
5. The facility's Hazard Communication Program.
6. Manufacturers' Material Safety Data Sheets for chemicals used in the facility.
7. Manufacturers' instructions for operating all equipment used in the facility.

Chapter Summary

1. OSHA requires employers to have an Exposure Control Plan and to provide free training, during working hours, about occupational exposure to bloodborne pathogens and hazardous chemicals.

2. A health care facility Infection Control Manager is responsible for maintaining and implementing the Exposure Control Plan and, at the least, assuring employees' compliance with other infection control procedures.

3. To avoid inappropriate job placement, new employees should have health inventories and any necessary physical examinations and laboratory tests before starting work.

4. All employees (permanent and contractual) must be retrained each year and when new occupational exposure risks occur.

5. Among the subjects that must be covered in the OSHA-required training program are explanations of: (a) the epidemiology and symptoms of bloodborne diseases; (b) the transmission routes of bloodborne pathogens; and (c) the uses and limitations of techniques to reduce exposure.

6. Employees must be trained in the use of hazardous chemicals before being exposed to them.

7. OSHA requires that training sessions be conducted by qualified individuals in a way comprehensible to all trainees.

8. Employees must have easy access to all required documents.

Chapter 10   Record Keeping

Accurate record keeping provides detailed evidence of the infection control measures described in previous chapters. In addition to the medical and training records described below, health care facilities must also continuously maintain documentation of sterilization monitoring results *[see Chapter 6, Monitoring Sterilization (Step 5)]* and regulated waste disposals made by haulers *(see Chapter 8, Disposal of Regulated Waste, item 1).*

Employee Medical Records

Table 27 describes OSHA-required, confidential, employee medical records.[23] In addition, the CDC recommends that tuberculin skin test results be recorded in health care workers' medical records and in an aggregate database of tuberculin skin test results for all health care workers.[3] Individual states and localities may have further requirements for medical record keeping and confidentiality.

OSHA Logs

Incorporated clinical practices and employers with more than 10 employees during the preceding calendar year must maintain the OSHA logs listed below. These logs do not substitute for the employee medical records described in Table 27.

Table 27. Confidential Employee Medical Records and OSHA Compliance

Requirements for employers:

1. Establish and maintain for each occupationally exposed employee an accurate medical record including:
   a. The employee's name and social security number.
   b. A copy of the employee's hepatitis B vaccination status, including the dates of all hepatitis B vaccinations and any medical records relative to an employee's ability to receive the vaccination.
   c. A copy of all results of postexposure examinations, <u>non</u>-blood medical testing, and follow-up procedures.
   d. The employer's copy of the health care professional's written opinion.
   e. A copy of the information provided to the health care professional *(see also Chapter 4, Table 5).*

2. Ensure that employee medical records are kept confidential and are not disclosed or reported, without an employee's express written consent, to anyone within or outside the workplace except as required by law.

3. Maintain an employee's required medical records for at least the duration of the employee's employment, plus 30 years.

4. Provide required employee medical records, upon request, for examination and copying, to an employee, anyone having written consent of an employee, the Director of the National Institute for Occupational Safety and Health, and the Assistant Secretary of Labor for Occupational Safety and Health (or any designated representatives of these officials).

Logs 300 and 301

Employers should use Log 300 to document occupational injuries and illness, and deaths related to either of these. *(See also: Sharps Injury Log.)* Health care workers in states and territories operating their own OSHA-approved programs *(see Appendix A)* should check applicable laws, because a few states still require <u>all</u> employers to maintain injury and illness records. Log 301 is used to document supplementary information on individual employees when worker's compensation or insurance reports, with similar data, have not been prepared.

Sharps Injury Log

Employers should use this log to record percutaneous injuries from contaminated sharps. The information shall be recorded and maintained in such manner as to protect the confidentiality of the injured employee. This log shall contain, at a minimum: (1) the type and brand of device involved in the incident; (2) the department or work area where the exposure incident occurred; and (3) an explanation of how the incident occurred. Further details on the requirements for this log, effective as of April 18, 2001, can be found in "Needlesticks and Other Sharps Injuries; Final Rule," *Federal Register,* 66(12):5318-5325, January 18, 2001. This is an addition to section 1910.1030(h) of OSHA's "Occupational Exposure to Bloodborne Pathogens; Final Rule."

Employers must keep all of the above logs for 5 years after the end of the year they cover, and make them available, for inspection and copying, to employees, former employees, and representatives of the Departments of Labor, and Health and Human Services.

Training Records

OSHA requires employers to keep employee bloodborne pathogen training records that include the:

1. Dates of the training sessions.

2. Contents or summaries of the training sessions.

3. Names and qualifications of persons conducting the training.

4. Names and job titles of all persons attending the training sessions.

Employers must maintain training records for 3 years from the date on which the training occurred. If employers cease to do business and there are no successor employers to receive and retain the records for the prescribed period, the employers must notify the Director of the National Institute for Occupational Safety and Health (NIOSH) at least 3 months prior to their disposal, and transmit them to the Director, if requested to do so, within that period. Employers must also, upon request, provide these employee training records for examination and copying to employees, employee representatives, the Director of NIOSH, and the Assistant Secretary of Labor for Occupational Safety and Health (or designated representatives of these officials).

Chapter Summary

1. OSHA requires employers to maintain documentation of: (a) sterilization monitoring results; and (b) regulated waste disposals made by haulers.

2. Employers must also maintain continuous records of employees': (a) medical conditions and evaluations; (b) occupational injuries; and (c) OSHA-required bloodborne pathogen training.

Definitions

Acquired immunodeficiency syndrome — a specific group of diseases or conditions that are indicative of severe immunosuppression related to infection with the human immunodeficiency virus (HIV).

Acute — pertaining to a process (i.e., a symptom, condition, or disease) with a rapid onset, severe symptoms, and a short course.

Acute retroviral syndrome — an illness characterized by fever, rash, myalgia, fatigue, malaise, or lymphadenopathy, which might be indicative of acute HIV infection, but also might be indicative of a drug reaction or another medical condition.

AIDS — acquired immunodeficiency syndrome.

Air/water syringe — a dental-unit device that can produce a stream or spray of air or water.

Alveolus (pl., alveoli) — an air sac in the lungs; found in clusters at the end of an alveolar duct.

Amniotic fluid — the fluid in the amnion.

Anaphylaxis — an immediate hypersensitive reaction to an allergen (e.g., a specific food or drug).

Antibiotic — a chemical substance (e.g., bacitracin, penicillin) produced by microorganisms, fungi, or synthetic means which, in dilute solution, can inhibit the growth of or kill other microorganisms.

Antibody — protein (immunoglobulin) manufactured by lymphocytes to neutralize or destroy antigen (foreign protein) in the body.

Antigen — a substance, such as a toxin, foreign protein, bacterium, or cell tissue, capable of inducing an immune response (i.e., stimulating production of an antibody).

Arthroscope — an endoscope used to examine the interior of a joint.

Aspergillus fumigatus — the yeastlike fungus that causes aspergillosis, marked by inflammatory lesions in the lungs, skin, ears, sinuses, and/or other body parts.

Asymptomatic — without symptoms.

Attenuated vaccine — a vaccine prepared from live microorganisms cultured under adverse conditions, leading to loss of their virulence but retention of their ability to induce protective immunity.

Bacteremia — the presence of bacteria in the blood.

Bacterial endospore — a dormant yet viable structure, formed inside rod-shaped bacteria (e.g., *Bacillus anthracis),* which can remain viable and potentially infectious for years. Bacterial endospores are extremely resistant to high temperatures and chemical agents; therefore, *Bacillus stearothermophilus* and *Bacillus subtilis* variety *niger* are often used to biologically monitor sterilization cycles.

Bactericidal — capable of destroying bacteria.

Bioaerosols — airborne droplets and droplet nuclei produced when people sneeze, cough, talk, or sing; mists generated when, for example, dental professionals use an air turbine handpiece or ultrasonic cleaner.

Biofilm — a surface attachment of live microorganisms forming a layer or mass.

Biohazard — refers to a potentially dangerous infectious agent; the word is used with a special symbol on warning labels affixed to regulated waste.

Bivalent vaccine — one containing two vaccine pathogens (e.g., both measles and rubella).

Bloodborne pathogen — a microbe, present in human blood, which can cause disease.

Blood plasma — the pale yellow liquid in which red and white blood cells and platelets are suspended.

Body Substance Isolation — body substance isolation; an infection control approach which considers all body substances from all patients to be pathogenic, whether or not the patients are diagnosed as infectious. *See Standard Precautions.*

Bronchiolitis — inflammation of the bronchioles, comprising small subdivisions (0.5 to 1 millimeter in diameter) of the bronchial tubes.

Bronchitis — inflammation of bronchial tube mucosa.

Bronchoscopy — the process of inserting a flexible fiberoptic tube into the tracheobronchial tree.

Bur — a dental drill bit with tungsten carbide steel edges or a coating of diamond grit.

Candida albicans — a yeast-like fungus that causes candidiasis, which most commonly involves the skin, oral mucosa, and vagina.

Carrier — a person harboring a pathogenic organism and capable of infecting others. Human carriers can be asymptomatic, incubatory, convalescent, and/or chronic.

Catarrh (adj., catarrhal) — mucous membrane inflammation, especially in the nose and throat.

CDC — Centers for Disease Control and Prevention, an agency of the U.S. Public Health Service; although the CDC does not have legal enforcement powers, it makes strong recommendations, based on current research in the health care field.

Cellulitis — an infection of subcutaneous or deeper tissues, resulting in acute, diffuse, edematous, and suppurative inflammation.

Cerebrospinal fluid — the fluid in the four ventricles of the brain and in the spinal cord's central canal.

Cervical — pertaining to the neck or the cervix.

Chemotherapy — treatment of an infection or disease by means of oral or injectable drugs.

Chickenpox (also: varicella) — a disease caused by the varicella zoster virus; marked by vesicles on the skin and mucous membranes and, in adults, possible complications of encephalitis or pneumonia.

Chronic — pertaining to a process (i.e., a symptom, condition, or disease) having a long course or recurring frequently.

Chuck — the gripping mechanism that holds a rotating tool.

Coccidioides immitis — the fungus that causes coccidioidomycosis, marked by acute respiratory infection.

Cohort — placing patients with the same diseases in the same hospital rooms.

Colitis — inflammation of the colon.

Colonization — the presence, growth, and proliferation of microorganisms in one or more body sites without producing observable clinical symptoms or immune reactions; often, the prelude to infection of the carrier and others.

Colostrum — milky, yellow fluid secreted by the mammary gland just before or after giving birth.

Congenital — present at or before birth (e.g., mental or physical traits or diseases, etc., which are hereditary or the result of something occurring during gestation).

Conjunctiva — the mucous membrane lining the inner surface of the eyelid and anterior part of the sclera, the white outer coat of the eyeball.

Conjunctivitis — inflammation of the conjunctiva, the mucous membrane lining the eyelids and covering the forepart of the sclera.

Contagion period — the time during which an infectious pathogen can be transmitted between humans.

Contaminated — carrying potentially infectious materials.

Contraindication — any condition that renders a particular line of treatment or prophylaxis improper or undesirable.

Creutzfeldt-Jakob disease — a rare, transmissible degenerative disease of the brain that occurs in middle life and is usually fatal.

Critical-class instrument or device — items that penetrate soft tissue, bone, or the vascular system, or allow blood to flow through them.

Cryptococcus neoformans — the fungus that causes cryptococcosis, marked by infection of the brain and meninges.

Cutaneous — pertaining to the skin.

Deoxyribonucleic acid — the main constituent of a cell's chromosomes; in all organisms except ribonucleic acid (RNA) viruses, it contains the genetic code.

Dermatitis — inflammation of the skin.

Disinfectant — a substance that destroys or inhibits the growth of disease-causing microbes, but not necessarily of all their forms (e.g., bacterial endospores).

Disseminated — widely scattered throughout an organ or the body.

DNA — deoxyribonucleic acid.

Droplet nuclei — minute particles remaining in the air after the water has evaporated from droplets emitted from the nose or mouth during sneezing and coughing.

Droplets — large (100 micrometers or more in diameter) droplets in respiratory tract secretions expelled by sneezing, coughing, or talking, or in saliva particles spattered during dental procedures.

Dry heat sterilizer — an instrument that sterilizes by means of heated air.

Eczema — inflammation of the skin, marked by erythema, papules, pustules, scabs, and/or vesicles.

Electrocardiographic lead — a conductor connecting a patient to an electrocardiograph, which makes graphic records of minute differences in electrical potential caused by heart-muscle action.

Encephalitis — inflammation of the brain.

Endocarditis — an inflammation of the endothelial membrane (endocardium) which lines the heart cavities.

Endogenous infection — an infection caused by pathogens already living inside the host.

Endoscope — an instrument used to examine the inside of large body organs such as the bladder.

Endospore — *see Bacterial endospore.*

Endotracheal intubation — insertion of a tube into the trachea to provide an airway or to allow administration of anesthesia and aspiration of secretions.

Enterococcus — a genus of Gram-positive bacteria; formerly, members of the genus *Streptococcus.*

Epidemic — a sudden, rapid spread of an infectious disease, simultaneously attacking many people in the same geographical area.

Exogenous infection — an infection caused by pathogens transmitted to a host from an outside source.

Extension cone — an open-ended, lead-lined cylinder that restricts an x-ray beam to the area being studied.

Fecal-oral transmission — the typical path of infection for hepatitis A and E (e.g., a person with fecal material containing the virus on his or her hands touches another person's food or drink, and the second person then ingests the virus.)

Gastroenteritis — inflammation of the stomach and intestines.

Gingival — pertaining to the gingiva or gums.

Glutaraldehydes — a group of liquid sterilants that should be used to sterilize only those semicritical instruments or materials that cannot tolerate exceptionally high temperatures.

Green soap — a potassium soap made from certain vegetable oils retaining glycerin.

Guillain-Barré syndrome — an acute, immune-mediated disorder affecting spinal roots and peripheral and cranial nerves.

Handpiece — a powered, hand-held device that engages rotary instruments used in surgeries.

HBsAg — *see Hepatitis B surface antigen.*

Health care worker — a person, including a student and trainee, who works or has worked in a health care, clinical, or medical laboratory setting.

Hemolytic uremic syndrome — a rare, acute illness marked by anemia, nephropathy, purpura, and thrombocytopenia; can be a complication of *Escherichia coli* serotype O157:H7 infection.

Hemostat — a surgical clamp used to compress a blood vessel to stop hemorrhaging.

HEPA (high-efficiency particulate air) filter — a specialized filter used in ventilation systems to remove tiny particles from the air or in personal respirators to filter air before it is inhaled.

Hepatitis, viral — an inflammation of the liver, caused by hepatitis viruses A, B, C, D, E, or G.

Hepatitis B surface antigen — the protein present on the outer surface of the hepatitis B virion.

Herpes zoster — a disease caused by recrudescence of latent varicella zoster virus infection; marked by severe neuralgic pain and clustered vesicles.

High-volume evacuation (also: high-speed or high-velocity air evacuation) — powerful vacuuming of an operating field.

Histoplasma capsulatum — the fungus that causes histoplasmosis, marked by a primary pulmonary lesion and, in AIDS patients, dissemination through the blood stream.

HIV — human immunodeficiency virus, the cause of AIDS.

Hydrogen peroxide, H_2O_2 — a colorless liquid used medically as a mild antiseptic and as a sterilant in a gas plasma sterilization process.

Hydrophilic virus — a virus that lacks a lipid, or water insoluble, envelope (e.g., adenoviruses, coxsackieviruses, and polioviruses); not destroyed by isopropyl alcohol.

Hyperbilirubinemia — an excessive amount of bilirubin in the blood.

Immune globulin — an antibody-containing solution derived from pooled human blood plasma; used to achieve passive immunization.

Immune system — a collection of cells and proteins that works to protect the body from potentially harmful infectious microorganisms, such as bacteria, viruses, and fungi.

Immunity — protection against a particular disease, generally provided by a previous infection or by vaccination.

Immunization — the process of inducing or providing immunity by any means, active or passive.

Immunocompetent — having the capacity to mount a normal immune response to an antigen.

Immunocompromised — having the immune response weakened by malnutrition, disease, irradiation, and/or administration of immunosuppressive drugs.

Immunoglobulin — one of a family of proteins (designated IgA, IgD, IgE, IgG, and IgM), some of which (but perhaps not all) may be capable of acting as antibodies. (All antibodies are immunoglobulins.)

Infection — the presence, growth, and proliferation of microorganisms in body tissues, usually followed by clinical signs (e.g., inflammation) that are not always apparent but can be identified by laboratory tests and/or other means.

Intubation — inserting a tube into a hollow anatomical structure (e.g., the larynx) to admit air or a fluid.

Invasive — refers to medical procedures that involve a skin incision or puncture, or insertion of an instrument into the body.

Iodophor — an iodine-based agent used to disinfect precleaned, noncritical-class devices; also used as an antimicrobial agent in certain hand-cleansing products.

Keratoconjunctivitis — inflammation of the cornea and conjunctiva.

Koplik's spots — blue-white spots which, on days 2 and 3 of measles, appear on the buccal mucosa opposite the molars, then spread to involve the entire buccal and labial mucosa.

Laparoscope — an endoscope used for visual examination of the peritoneal cavity.

Latent — present or potential, but not manifesting itself.

Lipophilic virus — a virus with a lipid, or water-insoluble, envelope (e.g., hepatitis B virus, herpes simplex virus, and human immunodeficiency virus).

Lymphangitis — inflammation of lymphatic vessels caused by bacterial infection.

Material Safety Data Sheet — a form manufacturers provide with each chemical sold, describing the product's dangers and the necessary safety measures.

Meningitis — infection of the meninges (the three membranes that envelope the brain and spinal cord). Meningitis can be caused by a variety of pathogens, including *Neisseria meningitidis* and *Streptococcus pneumoniae*.

Meningococcus — *Neisseria meningitidis.*

Microbe — *see Pathogen.*

Micrometer (μm; micron) — a unit of measure that equals 0.000001 meter.

MMR — measles-mumps-rubella (vaccine).

Monovalent vaccine — a vaccine containing antigens from only one strain of microorganism.

Mucous membrane (also: mucosa) — a membrane lining all bodily passages open to the air (e.g., parts of the digestive and respiratory tracts).

Multidrug-resistant tuberculosis — active tuberculosis caused by *Mycobacterium tuberculosis* organisms that are resistant to more than one anti-tuberculosis drug.

Mycobacteria (also: acid-fast bacteria) — Gram-positive bacteria of the genus *Mycobacterium;* these bacteria retain certain dyes after being washed in an acid solution

Nasopharynx (adj., nasopharyngeal) — that portion of the pharynx above the soft palate; it is continuous with the nasal passages.

Necrotizing fasciitis (also: hemolytic streptococcal gangrene; "flesh-eating" condition) — an infection usually caused by *Streptococcus pyogenes,* or a combination of bacteria; marked at first by severe cellulitis, which then spreads to the superficial and deep fascia (fibrous tissue), where thrombosis of subcutaneous vessels can lead to gangrene of the underlying tissues.

Negative pressure — the difference in relative air-pressure between two areas in a health care facility. A room at negative pressure has a lower pressure than adjacent areas, thereby keeping air from flowing out of the room.

Neonate — a newborn infant.

NIOSH — National Institute for Occupational Safety and Health of the CDC.

Noncritical-class device — equipment that contacts intact skin but not mucosa.

Nosocomial infection — an infection manifested after an admitted patient has been in a hospital for 72 hours or soon after the patient is discharged.

Occupational exposure — exposure to a bloodborne pathogen during the performance of an employee's duties. OSHA also uses the term to describe risk of occupational exposure: the reasonably anticipated skin, eye, mucous membrane, or parenteral contact with blood or other potentially infectious materials.

OSHA — Occupational Safety and Health Administration, a federal agency whose standards must be met by specified private-sector employers. (Part of the Department of Labor.)

Otitis media — inflammation of the middle ear.

Outbreak — a sudden increase in disease incidence in one specific area.

Pandemic — prevalent worldwide; an epidemic affecting many people in different countries.

Parenteral — pertaining to introduction of substances to the body by means other than through the gastrointestinal tract (e.g., intravenous, subcutaneous, or intramuscular).

Parotitis — inflammation of a parotid gland.

Paroxysm — 1. a sudden attack, recurrence, or intensification of symptoms of a disease. 2. a sharp spasm or convulsion of any kind.

Pathogen — a microbe (e.g., bacterium, virus, fungus, parasitic protozoan) capable of infecting a susceptible host and causing disease.

PEP — postexposure prophylaxis.

Peracetic acid (also: peroxyacetic acid), CH_3CO-O-OH — acetic acid plus an extra oxygen atom, which destroys pathogen cells; the chemical is used as a sterilant in the Steris System 1™.

Percutaneous — effected or performed through the skin (e.g., an injury to the skin or the injection, removal, or absorption of a substance via the skin).

Pericardium (adj., pericardial) — the fluid-filled membranous sac surrounding the heart.

Perinatal — around the time of birth.

Peritoneum (adj., peritoneal) — the membrane lining the abdominopelvic walls.

Personal protective equipment — specialized clothing or equipment (e.g., examination and utility gloves, gowns, masks, lab coats, foot wear, and face shields or goggles) worn as protection against a hazard.

Pharyngitis — inflammation of the pharynx.

Phenolic — a phenol-based chemical disinfectant.

Plebotomy — the process of opening a vein, via needle puncture or incision, to withdraw or let out blood.

Pleura (adj., pleural) — the thin serous membrane that enfolds the lungs and lines the chest cavity.

Pneumococcus — *Streptococcus pneumoniae.*

Pneumonia — a disease caused by bacteria, viruses, or fungi; marked by lung inflammation and exudate-filled air spaces.

PPD — purified protein derivative of tuberculosis, used as an intradermal skin test to screen for tuberculosis.

Prion — a small infectious, proteinaceous particle not susceptible to sterilization procedures which inactivate nucleic acids.

Prophylaxis — use of a drug, procedure, or type of equipment used to prevent disease.

Pulmonary — pertaining to the lungs.

Pumice — a rough, porous, grayish powder, used as a polishing agent.

Rag wheel — a cotton lathe attachment, used to smooth and polish prostheses.

Recombinant — gene-spliced genetic material.

Recrudesce — to renew activity following a latent period.

Regulated waste — as defined by OSHA: blood, other potentially infectious materials, or items contaminated with blood or other potentially infectious materials.

Resistance — the ability of some strains of bacteria to grow and multiply in the presence of certain drugs that ordinarily kill them; these strains are referred to as drug-resistant strains.

Rheumatic fever — a systemic, febrile, inflammatory, and nonsuppurative syndrome with varying severity, duration, and sequelae; often followed by serious heart or kidney disease and most frequently affecting children and young adults.

Rhinitis — inflammation of the nasal mucous membranes.

Ribonucleic acid — a nucleic acid that contains genetic instructions for the synthesis of proteins.

Risky sex — the act of having unprotected sexual contact with high-risk individuals (e.g., male homosexuals, injecting drug abusers, bisexual males, partners having extramarital sexual relations).

RNA — ribonucleic acid.

Rubber dam — rubber material temporarily placed on a dental patient's teeth to reduce saliva at the operative site and to minimize the pathogens in aerosols.

Scarlet fever — a disease caused by the group A streptococcus; marked by a characteristic rash lasting 6 to 9 days.

Semicritical-class instrument or device — items that do not meet critical-class criteria, but do contact either mucous membranes or broken skin. *See Critical-class instrument or device.*

Sepsis syndrome — a medical crisis, in which a weakened immune system releases substances causing deterioration of the patient's blood-vessel walls.

Seroconversion — the change of a serologic test from negative to positive, indicating the development of antibodies in response to infection or immunization.

Serologic — relating to the blood.

Seropositive — showing a significant level of serum antibodies.

Serotype — a microorganism distinguishable by its antigenicity from other strains in a species or subspecies.

Sharps — any objects capable of penetrating the skin (e.g., needles, broken glass).

Shingles — *see Herpes zoster.*

Source patient — a person, living or dead, whose blood or other potentially infectious body substances may expose a health care worker to infection.

Sputum — mucus or pus, mixed with saliva, coughed up from the lungs.

Standard Precautions — infection control guidelines, recommended by the CDC in 1996, which combine the major components of Universal Precautions and Body Substance Isolation.

***Staphylococcus* (pl., staphylococci; adj., staphylococcal)** — a genus of Gram-positive bacteria found on the skin of most humans. If skin or mucous membranes are disrupted, staphylococci may penetrate underlying tissues and the blood.

Sterilant — a chemical substance that totally destroys all microbial life forms, including viruses and spores.

Sterilization — the process of destroying all pathogens.

Strain — a group of organisms within a species, characterized by a particular quality.

***Streptococcus* (pl., streptococci; adj., streptococcal)** — a genus of Gram-positive bacteria; normal in humans but also associated with infections.

Syndrome — a group of symptoms and/or signs which together are characteristic of a specific disease or disorder.

Synergism (adj., synergistic) — a harmonious action of two drugs or chemicals, producing an effect which is greater than the total effects of each drug/chemical alone, or one that neither drug/chemical could produce alone.

Synovial fluid (also: synovia) — the lubricating fluid secreted by the synovium of a joint, bursa, or tendon sheath.

Systemic — affecting or pertaining to the whole body.

Thimerosal — a topical organic mercurial antiseptic, also used as a pharmaceutical preservative.

Thrombotic thrombocytopenic purpura — a rare disease marked by thrombosis and embolism of the brain's small blood vessels; can be a complication of *Escherichia coli* serotype O157:H7 infection.

Titer (or level) — the degree to which a substance may be diluted before it loses its ability to react with another substance. The term is associated with measurement of serum antibody levels.

Toxic shock syndrome — a severe illness mainly caused by infection with *Staphylococcus aureus,* and, sometimes, *Streptococcus pyogenes;* characterized by temperature of 102°F (38.9°C) or higher, a diffuse erythematous macular rash, hypotension, and multiple organ system disorders.

Toxoid — a bacterial toxin modified to be nontoxic but still able to stimulate the formation of an antitoxin.

Transmission-Based Precautions — CDC-recommended precautions to be used in addition to Standard Precautions when dealing with infections transmitted via specific routes (i.e., airborne, contact, and droplet).

Tuberculosis — an infectious disease, caused by *Mycobacterium tuberculosis,* that predominantly affects the lungs but is often found in other organs. The infection can be: (1) active and communicable (patients have signs, symptoms, and/or radiographic evidence of the disease); or (2) latent and noncommunicable (patients are asymptomatic but have dormant, viable *Mycobacterium tuberculosis* organisms in their granulomas).

Ultrasonic cleaner — a machine used to preclean instruments prior to sterilization.

Ultrasonic scaler — a dental instrument that aids in the removal of calcified plaque from tooth surfaces.

Universal Precautions — infection control procedures required by OSHA's bloodborne pathogen regulations.

Vaccination — the introduction of a vaccine or toxoid into the body to induce immunity to a specific infectious disease.

Vaccine — a suspension of whole or fractionated bacteria or viruses rendered nonpathogenic; administered to humans to induce immunity and prevent the diseases caused by the various bacteria or viruses.

Vesicle — a small, slightly elevated, fluid-filled sac which develops on skin or mucous membranes.

Virus — a metabolically inert pathogen able to replicate only within the cells of a living host.

Waterhouse-Friderichsen syndrome — an overwhelming bacteremia, the malignant form of cerebrospinal meningitis, characterized by the sudden onset of fever, coma, and circulatory collapse.

Appendix A   Information Sources

American Dental Association (ADA)
211 E. Chicago Ave., Chicago, IL 60611
312-440-2500; fax 312-440-2800
www.ada.org

**Association for Professionals in
    Infection Control and Epidemiology
    (APIC)**
1275 K St., NW., Suite 1000, Washington,
    DC 20005-4006
202-789-1890; fax: 202-789-1899
www.apic.org

**Centers for Disease Control and
    Prevention (CDC)**
1600 Clifton Road, Atlanta, GA 30333
404-639-3311
www.cdc.gov
CDC hotline: 770-488-7100
CDC clinician information line:
877-554-4625

Food and Drug Administration (FDA)
5600 Fishers Lane, Rockville, MD 20857
888-463-6332
www.fda.gov

**National Institute of Allergy and
    Infectious Diseases (NIAID)**
Office of Communications
Building 31, Room 7A50, Bethesda, MD
    20892-2520
301-496-5717; fax: 301-402-1020
www.niaid.nih.gov

**Organization for Safety and Asepsis
    Procedures (OSAP)**
P.O. Box 6297, Annapolis, MD 21401
800-298-6727; fax: 410-571-0028
www.osap.org

**National Institute for Occupational
    Safety and Health (NIOSH), CDC**
200 Independence Ave., SW., Room 715H,
    Washington, DC 20201
800-356-4674; fax: 513-533-8573
www.cdc.gov/niosh/home page.html

Occupational Safety and Health Administration (OSHA)

Main Office: 200 Constitution Ave., NW, Washington, DC 20210
202-219-7242; emergency calls: 800-321-6742 and TTY: 877-889-5627
www.osha.gov

OSHA Region 1: CT,[†] MA, ME, NH, RI, VT[†]
JFK Federal Building, Room E340 , Boston, MA 02203
617-565-9860

OSHA Region 2: NJ,[†] NY,[†] PR,[†] VI[†]
201 Varick St., Room 670, New York, NY 10014
212-337-2378

OSHA Region 3: DC, DE, MD,[†] PA, VA,[†] WV
US Department of Labor/OSHA
Curtis Center, Suite 740 West, 170 South Independence Mall West,
Philadelphia, PA 19106-3309
215-861-4900

OSHA Region 4: AL, FL, GA, KY,[†] MS, NC,[†] SC,[†] TN[†]
61 Forsyth St., SW, Atlanta, GA 30303
404-562-2300.

OSHA Region 5: IL, IN,[†] MI,[†] MN,[†] OH, WI
230 S. Dearborn St., Room 3244, Chicago, IL 60604
312-353-2220

OSHA Region 6: AR, LA, NM,[†] OK, TX
525 Griffin St., Room 602, Dallas, TX 75202
972-850-4145

OSHA Region 7: IA, [†]KS, MO, NE
City Center Square, 1100 Main St., Suite 800, Kansas City, MO 64105
816-426-5861

OSHA Region 8: CO, MT, ND, SD, UT,[†] WY[†]
1999 Broadway, Suite 1690, Denver, CO 80202
720-294-6550

OSHA Region 9: American Samoa, AZ,[†] CA,[†] Guam, HI,[†] NV,[†] Trust Territories of the Pacific
71 Stevenson St., Room 420, San Francisco, CA 94105
415-975-4310

OSHA Region 10: AK,[†] ID, OR,[†] WA[†]
1111 Third Ave., Suite 715, Seattle, WA 98101-3212
206-553-5930

[†] These 26 states and territories operate their own OSHA-approved job safety and health programs; however, CT, NJ, NY, and VI plans cover public employees only.

Appendix B. Preexposure Vaccination Checklist for U.S. Residents

For complete information, readers should refer to vaccine package inserts and pharmaceutical texts.

Diseases/Vaccines	Recipients	Doses	Contraindications
Anthrax Inactivated cell-free anthrax vaccine	• Ages 18 to 65 *and potentially exposed to large amounts of the bacterium on the job (e.g., laboratory workers, veterinarians, and military personnel).*	• Six-dose primary series: first three doses at 2-week intervals; last three doses, each one 6 months after the previous dose. Annual booster doses are needed.	• Serious allergic reaction to a previous dose. • Recovery from cutaneous (skin) anthrax. • Pregnancy (consider vaccination for pregnant women who have been exposed, or are likely to be exposed, to *Bacillus anthracis*).
Chickenpox Live, attenuated varicella vaccine.	• Age 12 months to 18 months. • 13 years old and above. *Vaccine recipients should avoid salicylates for 6 weeks and pregnancy for 3 months.*	• One dose (infants). • Two doses 4 to 8 weeks apart (adolescents and adults).	• Documented evidence (physician diagnosis or serologic) of varicella infection. • Pregnancy or immunodeficiency. • Anaphylactic reaction to gelatin or neomycin. • Moderate or severe acute illness. • Receipt, within the previous 5 months, of antibody-containing blood products.
Diphtheria, tetanus, and pertussis Diphtheria and tetanus toxoids, combined with acellular pertussis vaccine (DTaP), for children under age 7. *See also Tetanus, Diphtheria, and Pertussis below.*	• Ages 2 months, 4 months, 6 months, 15 to 18 months, and 4 to 6 years old. (*Give fourth dose at age 12 months to 14 months if at least 6 months have elapsed since the third dose and the parents are unlikely to return the child to the clinic at age 15 months to 18 months.*)	• Five doses: • The four primary doses must be full standard doses (reduced doses may not provide adequate protection). • Give the fifth (booster) dose before children enter school if they received the four primary doses before their 4th birthday.	• Age 7 or older. • Severe allergic reaction to a primary dose. • Encephalopathy not due to a nonvaccine identifiable cause, within 7 days of vaccination. • Temperature of 105°F (40.6°C), persistent crying for 3 or more hours, or a hypotonic or hypotensive hyporesponsive episode within 48 hours of vaccination. • Convulsion within 3 days of vaccination. *When pertussis vaccine is contraindicated, use diphtheria-tetanus (DT) toxoids.*

Appendix B. Preexposure Vaccination Checklist for U.S. Residents (Continued)

For complete information, readers should refer to vaccine package inserts and pharmaceutical texts.

Diseases/Vaccines	Recipients	Doses	Contraindications
Haemophilus influenzae **type B** **infection** Conjugate vaccine.	• Ages 2 months, 4 months, 6 months (depending on brand used), and 12 months to 15 months.	• Three to four doses: first dose, plus one or two more primary doses (depending on the brand), and one booster dose (all brands).	• Hypersensitivity to any vaccine component. • Febrile illness.
Hepatitis A Inactivated vaccine.	• Age 2 to 12 years *and* living in areas with high case rates, and any travelers to such localities. • Food handlers, when health authorities or private employers deem vaccination to be beneficial. • Injecting drug abusers. • Men who have sex with men. • Persons with clotting-factor disorders or chronic liver disease. • Potentially exposed laboratory workers.	• Two doses: one primary dose and a booster dose 6 to 12 months later.	• Severe reaction to a prior hepatitis A vaccine dose. • Pregnancy (use the vaccine only when clearly needed).
Hepatitis B Recombinant vaccine.	• Infants through 18 years old (first check records for receipt of previous doses). *Infants under 6 months old should, preferably, receive vaccine not containing thimerosal.* • All health care workers and others who could be occupationally exposed to the virus. • Persons requiring hemodialysis or frequent blood transfusions or clotting factor concentrate receipt. • International travelers. • Persons whose lifestyles (e.g., illicit drugs or risky sex) may expose them to the virus.	• Three dose series: the first two doses 4 weeks apart; the third dose, *at least 2 months after second* dose. *Infants born to HBsAg-positive (or unknown status) mothers should receive the first dose within 12 hours of birth and complete the series by age 6 months.*	• Anaphylactic reaction to yeast or any component of the vaccine. • Multiple sclerosis (consider possible disease exacerbation versus benefits of vaccination).

Appendix B. Preexposure Vaccination Checklist for U.S. Residents (Continued)

For complete information, readers should refer to vaccine package inserts and pharmaceutical texts.

Disease/Vaccine	Recipients	Doses	Contraindications
Influenza Inactivated trivalent vaccine formulated for the current influenza season and administered annually during mid-October to mid-November. *Use split-virus vaccine for children under 13 years old.*	• Persons at high risk for influenza-related complications and severe disease, including • All children 6 to 59 months old. • Pregnant women. • Anyone age 50 or older. • Persons of any age with certain chronic medical conditions. • Persons who live with or care for persons at high risk, including • Household contacts who have frequent contact with persons at high risk. • Health care workers. • Age 6 months to 18 years old if receiving long-term aspirin therapy. • Persons who provide essential community services (e.g., police and fire department personnel). • Residents of nursing homes and other chronic-care facilities. • Persons who have required regular medical follow-up or hospitalization during the preceding year because of chronic metabolic disease (including diabetes mellitus), renal dysfunction, hemoglobinopathies, or immunosuppression. *Other persons age 6 months or older (e.g., HIV-infected persons, breastfeeding mothers, dormitory-residing students, military personnel, and persons traveling in large tourist groups or to the tropics) should be considered for vaccination.*	• One dose. *Children under age 9, who are receiving the vaccine for the first time, should receive two doses 4 weeks apart.*	• Moderate or serious acute, febrile illness. • Hypersensitivity to eggs, sodium bisulfite, or thimerosal. • Development of Guillain-Barré syndrome within 6 weeks of a previous influenza vaccination (when such persons are at high risk for influenza-related complications, consider vaccination).

Appendix B. Preexposure Vaccination Checklist for U.S. Residents (Continued)

For complete information, readers should refer to vaccine package inserts and pharmaceutical texts.

Diseases/Vaccines	Recipients	Doses	Contraindications
Measles (rubeola), mumps, and rubella (German measles) Preferably trivalent measles-mumps-rubella (MMR) vaccine, although separate vaccines are available against each virus.	• Between ages 12 months and 15 months and at 4 to 6 years old. • Persons who can become pregnant or are at increased risk of acquiring *any* of the three diseases (e.g., susceptible health care workers, international travelers, and students entering college). • Persons vaccinated before their first birthday, or with killed measles vaccine during 1963-1967, an unknown vaccine type, or strains other than Edmonston B.	• Two doses: • Infants who receive the first dose even 1 day before age 12 months must restart the vaccination series. Although the second dose is usually given at ages 4 to 6 years old, it can be given earlier if at least 4 weeks have elapsed since receipt of the first dose and no doses were administered before age 12 months. • All health care workers lacking reliable documentation (*right*) should receive two doses 4 weeks apart. • All persons susceptible to any of the three diseases should receive two doses 4 weeks apart. (Persons born before 1957 can be given one dose if not able to become pregnant and not at increased risk.)	• Existence of documented: 1. Serologic evidence of immunity to measles, mumps, and rubella, or 2. Receipt of live virus vaccine against the infections on or after first birthday (i.e., two doses of measles vaccine; one dose of mumps and rubella vaccines), or 3. Physician-diagnosed infection (acceptable for measles and mumps *only* because many rash-causing illnesses mimic rubella infection). • Pregnancy or possibility of becoming pregnant within 3 months. Women identified as susceptible during pregnancy can be vaccinated in the immediate postpartum period. • Anaphylactic reaction to gelatin or neomycin (for patients allergic to eggs, use published protocols). • Immunodeficiency (except HIV-infected patients who are asymptomatic or are not severely immunosuppressed). • Moderate or severe acute illnesses. • Receipt, within the previous month, of large daily doses of corticosteroids for 14 days or more. • Receipt of antibody-containing blood products; the length of delay before MMR vaccination varies with the product.

Appendix B. Preexposure Vaccination Checklist for U.S. Residents (Continued)

For complete information, readers should refer to vaccine package inserts and pharmaceutical texts.

Diseases/Vaccines	Recipients	Doses	Contraindications
Meningococcal meningitis Polysaccharide quadrivalent (A, C, Y, and W-135) vaccine.	• Health care workers exposed to the bacterium in laboratories and/or working in areas where three or more confirmed or probable serogroup C cases occur in the course of 3 months or less. • Persons with asplenia or terminal complement deficiency. • Military recruits and travelers to areas where the infection is epidemic (see www.cdc.gov/travel).	• One dose. *Inform dormitory-residing college freshmen that the vaccine could reduce their risks of infection.*	• Pregnancy. • Acute illness. • Less than 2 years old.
Pneumococcal pneumonia and meningitis • 7-valent pneumococcal conjugate vaccine (**PCV**). • 23-valent pneumococcal polysaccharide vaccine (**PPV**).	• Under 24 months old (**PCV**). • Ages 24 months to 59 months, if they have not received the vaccine *and* are at high risk for invasive *Streptococcus pneumoniae* infection (**PCV** or **PPV**). • Ages 2 to 64, if they: (1) are alcohol dependent or immunocompromised; (2) have asplenia, cardiomyopathies, chronic obstructive pulmonary disease, cirrhosis, congestive heart disease, diabetes, emphysema, or sickle cell anemia; or (3) live in nursing homes or other long-term-care facilities (**PPV**). Such persons can receive one revaccination if they are age 11 or older *and* 5 years have elapsed since their primary vaccination, or if they are age 10 or younger *and* 3 years have elapsed since the primary dose. • Age 65 or older: a **PPV** primary dose if they have never received the vaccine, or have unknown vaccination status. Persons in this age group can receive one revaccination if they received the vaccine when under 65 years old *and* 5 years have elapsed since the primary vaccination.	• One dose. *Also consider giving one PCV dose to children: (1) aged 24 to 35 months, (2) of Alaska Native, American Indian, or African-American descent, and (3) attending group day-care centers.* • One revaccination dose for certain persons *(see indications at left).*	• Acute respiratory or other active infection, unless lack of vaccination could present a greater risk.

Appendix B. Preexposure Vaccination Checklist for U.S. Residents (Continued)

For complete information, readers should refer to vaccine package inserts and pharmaceutical texts.

Diseases/Vaccines	Recipients	Doses	Contraindications
Poliomyelitis Inactivated poliovirus vaccine (IPV).	• Age 2 months, 4 months, 6 months to 18 months, and 4 to 6 years old. • Health care workers in close contact with patients excreting the virus or working with laboratory poliovirus specimens. • Travelers to endemic poliomyelitis areas.	• Four doses: three primary doses at each age *(left)* for infants and one booster dose for 4 to 6 year-olds. • Three doses for unvaccinated at-risk adults *(see left)*: two doses 4 to 8 weeks apart; third dose, 6 to 12 months after second dose. • One dose for at-risk adults who had previously received all three doses.	• Pregnancy. • An anaphylactic reaction to neomycin, streptomycin, or polymyxin B. • Moderate or severe acute febrile illness.
Smallpox Vaccine made from vaccinia virus.	• Unvaccinated health care workers engaged in research projects on vaccinia virus.	• One dose: normally every 10 years, but, if a case of smallpox is diagnosed, within 4 days of exposure.	• Pregnancy. • Immunodeficiency. • Active eczema.
Tetanus, diphtheria, and pertussis Tetanus-diphtheria-pertussis (Tdap) vaccine. *(See also Diphtheria, tetanus, and pertussis above.)*	• Age 7 and older if they did not receive the primary DTaP series *(see above)*. • Age 11 to 12 years old: booster Tdap dose if more than 5 years have elapsed since last primary dose.	• Three doses for primary series: 2 doses 4 weeks apart, third dose, 6 to 12 months later. • One booster dose: (1) at age 11 to 12 *(see left)*; and (2) for all persons, every 10 years *(sooner if an injury or intimate diphtheria exposure occur)*.	• Pregnancy (first trimester). • Severe local reactions to doses received within the past 10 years. • Acute infection (except for an emergency dose).
Tuberculosis Bacille Calmette-Guérin vaccine (BCG).	• Certain infants *(see right)*. • Health care workers employed in areas where multidrug-resistant tuberculosis is prevalent and infection control has failed to prevent transmission of the mycobacterium to such workers.	• One dose: • Tuberculin-negative infants who cannot be separated from patients with active pulmonary tuberculosis and cannot be given long-term tuberculosis therapy. • Health care workers *(left)*; first consult with health department on advisability.	• Pregnancy. • Immunodeficiency.

Appendix C. Infection Control Checklist for Outpatient Clinical Practices

M	T	W	Th	F	
					Open the office and make the clinical facility fully functional
					• Prepare "critical" inventory: personal protective equipment, disinfectants, antimicrobial soap, and other items for the day.
					• Clean sterilizer to receive instruments as used.
					• Make fresh holding solutions.
					Prepare for the first patient
					• Check treatment area cleanliness to make sure that night cleaning created no contamination; correct as necessary.
					• Disinfect treatment surfaces.
					• Put disposable (single-use) covers on fixtures.
					• Prepare treatment items (personal barriers, fresh sterile supplies).
					Manage the between-patients process
					• Create a smooth flow of repetitively used items.
					• Repeat step-by-step instrument preparation process all day.
					• Follow a between-patients checklist covering:
					• Removal of contaminated materials.
					• Cleaning and disinfection of contaminated surfaces.
					• Flushing of dental unit water lines.
					• Replacement of single-use items.
					• Availability of personal protective equipment.

Appendix C. Infection Control Checklist for Outpatient Clinical Practices (Continued)

M	T	W	Th	F	Close the office
					• Clean, package (if necessary), and sterilize contaminated items. (Do not wait until the next morning, since blood serum and debris can dry on items overnight.)
					• Clean and disinfect office and operatories. (Do not put out items that could be contaminated overnight.)
					• Complete other routines.
					• Empty, clean, and refill ultrasonic cleaner.

Weekly Infection Control Routines

					• Maintain checklists to document regulatory compliance.
					• Monitor publications for safety information.
					• Communicate with patients and staff on safety.
					• Supervise handling of contaminated laundry.
					• Maintain supplies, records, and training.
					• Process biological monitors at least weekly.
					• Disinfect dental unit water lines at least weekly.

PHOTO COPY THIS CHART AND CHECK OFF TO MAINTAIN ROUTINES

Appendix D Disease Spread in Dental Offices

Pathway 1: Dental Personnel to Patients

Spread of bloodborne and non-bloodborne agents from dental personnel to patients must involve the following:

- The dental staff member must be viremic (i.e., have virus particles present in the blood).

- The dental staff member must have a condition (e.g., weeping dermatitis or an injury) that allows direct exposure to his or her blood or other bodily fluid.

- The dental staff member's activity must allow his or her blood or another bodily fluid to gain direct access to a patient's wound, traumatized tissue, mucous membrane, or similar portal of entry.

Prevention
- Wear gloves and a mask, and avoid sharps injuries.

Work Restrictions
- Exclusion from duty:
  Measles (active or exposed if susceptible)
  Meningococcal infection
  Mumps (active or exposed if susceptible)

Whooping cough (pertussis)
Rubella (active, or exposed if susceptible)
Tuberculosis (active)
Chickenpox (active, or exposed if susceptible)

- <u>Restriction from patient contact:</u>
Conjunctivitis
Diarrheal disease (active)
Hepatitis A
Herpes infection on hands (herpetic whitlow)
Lice (pediculosis)
Staphylococcus aureus infection (draining skin lesions)
Group A staphylococcal infection
Shingles

Pathway 2: Patients to Dental Personnel (Bloodborne)

Hepatitis B
- Hepatitis B virus is transmitted by percutaneous or mucosal exposure to bodily fluids.

Hepatitis C
- Hepatitis C virus is not transmitted very efficiently through occupational exposures to blood and is not considered an occupational disease of dentistry. Most cases are a result of illegal drug use.

Hepatitis D
- Hepatitis D exists only in the presence of hepatitis B.

Human Immunodeficiency Virus (HIV)
- The risk of HIV infection among dental personnel is extremely low.

Overall Prevention
- Maintain appropriate immunizations for dental personnel.
- Avoid exposure to patients' oral fluids by practicing infection control procedures with regard to: PPE, sharps, operatory cleanup, instrument processing, laboratory work, and waste disposal.

Pathway 3: Patients to Other Patients

Potential causes:
- Improperly prepared instruments
- Contaminated clinical contact surfaces

Prevention
- Infection control procedures, including: PEP, cleaning and sterilizing instruments, and cleaning and disinfecting clinical contact surfaces.

Adapted from CDC guidelines for infection control in dental health-care settings.[9]

Index

acetone, 106
acquired immunodeficiency
    syndrome, 26, 64
acute respiratory disease, 55
adenovirus infection, 55, 57
air
    arid, and invading
        pathogens, 25
    filtration, 93
    pathogen transmission in,
        23
air/water syringe
    tip, 101
Airborne Precautions
    chickenpox/varicella and
        disseminated herpes
        zoster, 72
    description, 28, 29
    *Mycobacterium
        tuberculosis*, 42, 43
    rubeola virus
        infection/measles, 71
airborne transmission, 23
alcohol, 87, 106, 119
alcohol-based hand rub, 85
allergy
    alert card, 91
    latex, 90, 91
amalgam

and mercury, 103, 137
    condenser, 101
amantadine/rimantadine
    resistance, 14
American Dental
    Association, 99, 101, 125,
    137, 161
American Heart Association,
    16
amniotic fluid, and herpes
    simplex virus, 63
anaphylaxis, 91
anesthesia breathing circuit,
    118
anthrax, 34
antibody
    -containing blood
        products, 73
    to HBsAg, 59, 60
    to hepatitis C, 61
    to varicella, 72
antimetabolites, and
    Staphylococcus aureus
    infection, 48
antimicrobial
    agent in hand-cleansing
        product, 85, 87
    mouthrinse, 96
antitoxin, botulinum, 37

arthritis, and rubella virus
    infection, 70
arthroscope, 101
Aspergillus fumigatus, 16
Association for Professionals
    in Infection Control and
    Epidemiology, 81, 117,
    161
asthma, 25, 91
asymptomatic
    diphtheria carriers, 38
    hepatitis C virus infection,
        61
    pathogen colonization,
        123
    pneumococcus carriers,
        49
    Streptococcus pyogenes
        carriers, 50
autoclave, 105, 106
    Bowie-Dick test, 113
    drying cycle, 113
    loading, 109
    spore strip placement,
        111
    tape, 109
    treating regulated waste,
        136

autoinoculation, herpes
   simplex virus, 63
Bacille Calmette Guérin
   vaccine, 44
Bacillus
   anthracis
      infection, 14, 34
      resistance to heat or
         chemicals, 100
   stearothermophilus, 111
   subtilis, 111
bacteremia
   Staphylococcus aureus
      infection, 48
   Streptococcus
      pneumoniae infection,
      49
bacterial
   endocarditis, 16
   endospore, 104, 111, 112,
      118, 119
   filter, 114
   filtration efficiency, 93
bassinet, and phenolics, 119
bedpan disinfection, 119
bile, and hepatitis B virus, 58
bioaerosol
   Clostridium botulinum, 36
   cloud, variola virus, 73
   hazard, 31
biohazard warning label,
   OSHA-required, 135
biological
   monitoring, 110, 111
   safety cabinet, 18
bioterrorism hotline, CDC, 74
bleach. *See* sodium
   hypochlorite
blood
   coagulation, 107
   postexposure testing, 80
   pressure cuff disinfection,
      119
   splash, 29, 61, 77, 78
   transfusion, 25
blood containing
   cytomegalovirus, 57
   hepatitis A virus, 57

hepatitis B virus, 58
hepatitis C virus, 61
hepatitis G virus, 62
human immunodeficiency
   virus, 63
Mycobacterium
   tuberculosis, 41
Toxoplasma gondii, 51
bloodborne pathogens and
   occupational exposure,
   17, 79, 80
   OSHA-required training,
   144
Body Substance Isolation,
   27
boil water advisory, 124
bone
   chisel, 101
   spicule, 77
Bordetella pertussis
   infection, 35
botulism, 36
Bowie-Dick test, 113
breast milk containing
   cytomegalovirus, 56
   hepatitis B virus, 58
   human immunodeficiency
      virus, 63
bronchiolitis, and respiratory
   syncytial virus infection,
   69
bronchoscopy, 92, 123
bur, 108, 114, 128
   surgical, 101
burn unit patient, 26
Candida albicans, 16
   resistance to heat or
      chemicals, 100
carbon steel, 101, 107
cardiac disease, high-risk
   host, 25
cardiothoracic surgery, 26
case reporting
   acquired
      immunodeficiency
      syndrome, 66
   adenovirus infection, 56
   chickenpox, 73

Chlamydia pneumoniae
   infection, 36
Clostridium botulinum
   infection, 37
cryptosporidiosis, 39
diphtheria, 39
Escherichia coli infection,
   40
giardiasis, 41
hepatitis A, 58
hepatitis B, 61
herpes simplex virus
   infection, 63
human immunodeficiency
   virus infection, 66
influenza, 67
legionellosis, 41
measles (rubeola), 72
meningococcal meningitis,
   46
mumps, 68
Mycoplasma pneumoniae
   infection, 45
pertussis/whooping
   cough, 36
pneumococcal disease,
   49
poliomyelitis, 69
respiratory syncytial virus
   infection, 70
rubella/German measles,
   71
salmonellosis, 47
shigellosis, 47
smallpox, 74
Streptococcus pyogenes
   infection, 50
toxoplasmosis, 51
tuberculosis, 45
cat feces containing
   Toxoplasma gondii, 51
catarrhal stage, 35
catheter
   cardiac, 101
   indwelling urethral, 26
   insertion site disinfection,
      22
   intravascular, 15

cell-mediated immunity, 25
cellulitis, 50
Centers for Disease Control
  and Prevention, 161
  guidelines, 14
  Standard Precautions, 27
  Transmission-Based
    Precautions, 28
centrifuge, 18
cephalosporin, 49
cerebrospinal fluid
  containing hepatitis B
    virus, 58
cervical secretions
  containing
    cytomegalovirus, 56
chain of events, 114
chemical
  hazardous, 136. *See*
    Hazard
    Communication;
    Material Safety Data
    Sheet
  monitoring, sterilizer, 112
  vapor, unsaturated, 103
chemotherapy, 26
chickenpox/varicella, 29, 30
Chlamydia pneumoniae
  infection, 36
chloramine-T, 118
chlorhexidine, 85, 87
chronic
  disease, high-risk host, 25
  hepatitis B, 62
  obstructive pulmonary
    disease, 67, 70
cigarette smoker
  and influenza, 66
  and pneumonia, 36, 41,
    45, 49, 56
cilia, respiratory tract, 25
clinical surface disinfection,
  121
Clostridium botulinum
  infection, 36
  resistance to heat or
    chemicals, 100
Clostridium difficile, 84

Clostridium difficile infection,
  37
clothing
  OSHA requirements, 97
  protective, 96, 97, 106
clotting factor disorder, and
  hepatitis A virus, 57
Coccidioides immitis, 16
cohorting patients, 26, 73
cold sore, 63
colitis, 39
colonization, *Staphylococcus
  aureus*, 87
colostrum containing human
  immunodeficiency virus,
  63
common vehicle
  transmission, 24
communicating with patients,
  145
congenital
  rubella syndrome, 70
  toxoplasmosis, 51
  varicella syndrome, 72
conjunctivitis, 91. *See*
  keratoconjunctivitis
contact
  dermatitis, 91
  lenses, 98
  transmission, definition,
    24
  urticaria syndrome, 91
Contact Precautions
  adenoviruses, 56
  Clostridium difficile, 37
  congenital rubella
    syndrome, 70
  *Corynebacterium
    diphtheriae*, 38
  Cryptosporidium parvum,
    39
  description, 29, 30
  Escherichia coli, 40
  Giardia lamblia, 40
  hepatitis A virus, 57
  herpes simplex virus, 63
  norovirus, 68

respiratory syncytial virus,
  69
Salmonella, 46
Shigella sonnei, 47
Staphylococcus aureus,
  48
Streptococcus pyogenes,
  50
  vancomycin-resistant
    enterococcus, 51
container, regulated waste,
  134
corticosteroid, 26
Corynebacterium diphtheriae
  infection, 38
cosmetics, 98
coughing, and infection
  control, 43, 50, 69
coverings, protective, 121
Creutzfeldt-Jakob disease,
  103
critical-class instrument or
  device, 100, 101, 102,
  104
crutches, disinfection, 119
cryosurgical instrument, 101,
  118
Cryptococcus neoformans,
  16, 24
  resistance to heat or
    chemicals, 100
cryptosporidiosis, 39
Cryptosporidium parvum
  infection, 39
cutaneous
  anthrax, 34
  exposure, 77
cycle of infection, 21
  entry portal, 25
  exit vehicle, 22
  reservoir, 22
  susceptible host, 25
  transmission mode, 23
cytomegalovirus infection, 56
daylight loader, 122
defenses, human, 25
dental
  impression, 125

lathe unit, 125
radiographic equipment, 126
unit water line, 124
dentures, 125
Department of Veterans Affairs, 111
dermatitis, 84, 91
diabetes
and influenza, 66
high-risk host, 25
diaphram-fitting ring, 101
diphtheria, 38
direct contact transmission, 24
disinfection
high-level, 118
intermediate-level, 118
low-level, 118
disposal of regulated waste, 133
doorknob contamination, 24
dosimeter, 137
double-gloving, 91
droplet
infectious, large, 24, 95
nuclei, 23, 28, 41, 94, 95
transmission, 24
Droplet Precautions
adenoviruses, 56
Bordetella pertussis, 35
Corynebacterium diphtheriae, 38
description, 29
influenza viruses, 66
mumps virus, 67
Mycoplasma pneumoniae, 45
Neisseria meningitidis, 45
rubella, 70
Streptococcus pyogenes, 50
drug-resistant pathogen, 14, 66, 84. *See also* multidrug-resistant
dry heat sterilant, 102, 103
dust, infectious, 23, 28
eating restriction, 98

eczema, 63, 74, 91
electrocardiographic lead disinfection, 119
emerging and re-emerging infections, 14
employee
complaint, 138
free hepatitis B vaccine, 59
health inventory, 142
medical records, 147, 148
postexposure prophylaxis, 80
training, 142, 145
training records, 149
encephalitis and
measles, 71
Toxoplasma gondii, 51
West Nile virus, 25
endocarditis, 16
endogenous infection, 22
endoscope/endoscopy, 92, 123
endospore. *See* bacterial endospore
endotracheal tube, 118
engineering controls, 128
enterococci drug resistance, 14, 29, 30
vancomycin-resistant enterococcus (VRE), 51
entry portal. *See* cycle of infection
Environmental Protection Agency, 119, 121
Escherichia coli infection, 39
ethylene oxide, 102, 104
evacuation line, 136
examination gloves, 90
exit vehicle. *See* cycle of infection
exogenous infection, 22
Exposure Control Plan, 140, 144, 145
exposure-prone invasive procedure, 58, 64
extension cone, 122

eye
protection, 69, 88, 92, 95, 106
secretions, and adenovirus, 55
eyeglasses, 92, 95
eyewash station, 78
face mask. *See* mask
face shield, 92, 95
faucet contamination, 24
fecal-oral transmission, 57, 62
feces containing
Cryptosporidium parvum, 39
cytomegalovirus, 56
Escherichia coli, 39
Giardia lamblia, 40
hepatitis A virus, 57
hepatitis B virus, 58
hepatitis E virus, 62
poliovirus, 68
Salmonella, 46
Shigella sonnei, 47
Federal Bureau of Investigation, 34, 37, 74
fetal infection
cytomegalovirus, 56
Mycobacterium tuberculosis, 41
rubella virus, 70
rubeola virus, 71
Toxoplasma gondii, 51
varicella zoster virus, 72
fingernail care, 84
first aid, immediate, 78
fit-check, personal respirator, 94
flash sterilization, 101
flesh-eating disease, 50
Food and Drug Administration, 161
food containing
Clostridium botulinum, 36
Escherichia coli, 39
hepatitis A virus, 24, 57
poliovirus, 68
Salmonella, 24, 46

Shigella sonnei, 24, 47
Streptococcus pyogenes, 50
Toxoplasma gondii, 51
forceps, 101, 109, 130
formaldehyde, 106
freon, 104
fungal infection, 17, 90
gas plasma sterilization, 104
gastric acid, 25
gastrointestinal anthrax, 34
German measles. *See* rubella virus
Giardia lamblia infection, 40
giardiasis, 40
gloves
    double-gloving, 89
    examination, 90
    OSHA requirements, 89
    surgical, 90
    utility, 90
glutaraldehyde, 102, 104, 112, 113, 125
goggles, 92, 95
green soap, 126
hand
    antisepsis, 29, 84, 85
    -cleansing products, 87
    hygiene guidelines, 15
    -washing, 81
        after glove removal, 89
        OSHA-requirements, 82
        routine, 83
hand lotion, 84, 86
handling sterilized instruments, 113
handpiece, dental, 101, 108, 114
hazard
    controls, 128
    reporting, 138
Hazard Communication, 137, 143, 145
hazardous chemicals, preexposure training, 143
hemodialysis

hepatitis C virus infection, 61
preventing infection, 15
hemolytic uremic syndrome, 39
hemorrhagic colitis, 39
hemostat, 109, 130
HEPA personal respirator, 29, 34, 43, 93, 95
hepatitis A virus, 29
    in food, 24
    infection, 57
    postexposure prophylaxis, 57
hepatitis B virus
    e-antigen, 58
    infection, 58
    postexposure prophylaxis, 15, 60, 61
    resistance to heat or chemicals, 100
    surface antigen, 58, 62
hepatitis C virus
    infection, 61
    postexposure prophylaxis, 15
    postexposure testing, 62
hepatitis D, E, and G virus infection, 62
herpes
    labialis/genitalis, 63
    simplex virus, 63
    zoster (shingles), 29, 30, 72
herpetic whitlow, 63
high
    -efficiency particulate air respirator. *See* HEPA personal respirator
    -risk host, 25, 84
    -volume evacuation, 137
Histoplasma capsulatum, 16
hives, 91
hollow-bore needle, 61
homosexual, and hepatitis B, 58
housekeeping, 17, 120

human immunodeficiency virus
    infection, 63
    perinatal transmission, 16
    postexposure prophylaxis, 15, 64, 65
    resistance to heat or chemicals, 100
humoral immunity, 25
hydrogen peroxide, 102, 104
hydrophilic virus, 99
hyperbilirubinemia, 119
immediate first aid, 59, 61, 64, 78
immune globulin
    cytomegalovirus, 57
    hepatitis A, 57
    hepatitis B, 60
    rubeola, 71
    varicella, 73
immunization. *See* vaccine
impetigo, 50
implant, 101
implantable device, 101, 112
incubator, 111, 119
indirect contact transmission, 24
infant/neonate
    high-risk host, 26
    hyperbilirubinemia, 119
infection control checklist, 169
Infection Control Manager, 18, 29, 86, 140
inflammatory response, 25
influenza virus
    drug resistance, 14
    infection, 66
    preventing infection, 16
    prophylaxis against infection, 67
    transmission, 24, 29, 66
inhalation anthrax, 34
injecting drug use, illicit
    and hepatitis C, 61
    and hepatitis G virus, 62
injection, infectious, 77
inspection, OSHA, 138

integrator, 112
intensive-care unit
    patient, 26
intermediate-level
    disinfection, 118
intraabdominal surgery, 26
intravascular catheter
    infection, preventing, 15
intravenous insertion site, 25
intubation, 46, 92
invasive device. *See*
    catheter
invasive procedure,
    restriction, 58, 64
iodine, 119
iodophor, 85, 87, 119, 125
irrigation, 77
isolation
    guidelines, 26
    patient, 43
    precautions, 15
jaundice, hepatitis A, 57
Job Safety & Health
    Protection poster, 138
keratoconjunctivitis, 55
ketone, 106
kissing, open-mouthed, 24
laboratory worker and
    bloodborne pathogens, 17
    hepatitis A virus, 57
    Mycobacterium
        tuberculosis, 42
    Neisseria meningitidis, 46
laparoscope, 101
large-bore needle, 64
laryngotracheitis
    and measles, 71
latex
    allergy/hypersensitivity,
        90, 91, 142
    gloves, 90, 91
laundry, 96, 97
lead in radiograph film box,
    136
Legionella pneumophila
    infection, 41
legionellosis (Legionnaires'
    disease), 41

lesion secretions and
    Corynebacterium
        diphtheriae, 38
    Streptococcus pyogenes,
        50
lip balm, 98
lipid virus, 100
lipophilic virus, 100
liquid waste, 136
liver enzyme elevation,
    hepatitis A, 57
loading sterilizers, 109
logs, injury, OSHA-required,
    148
long-term care patient, 26
low-level disinfection, 119
lubricant, water-based, 106,
    108, 114
lymphangitis, 50
Mantoux tuberculin skin test,
    42, 44
mask. *See also* personal
    respirator
    OSHA requirement, 88,
        92
    surgical, 29, 30, 42, 43,
        45, 92, 95
Material Safety Data Sheet,
    137
measles (rubeola)
    Airborne Precautions, 29
    infection control, 29, 30
medical evaluation
    new employee, 142
    postexposure, 27, 80
meningitis and
    mumps, 67
    Neisseria meningitidis
        infection, 45
    Streptococcus
        pneumoniae infection,
        49
    West Nile virus, 25
meningococcal infection.
    See Neisseria
    meningitidis
    (meningococcus)
mercury, 103, 137

metal fragment, 77
methicillin. *See*
    Staphylococcus aureus
    drug resistance
microbe susceptibility, 99
military recruit, adenovirus
    infection, 56
mirror, oral, 101
monitoring sterilization, 110
mouth pipetting, 98
mouthrinse, 96
mouth-to-mouth
    resuscitation, 46, 94
mucosal exposure, 77
multidrug-resistant
    pathogen, Contact
    Precautions, 29, 30
mumps virus infection, 67
mycobacteria, 87, 118
Mycobacterium tuberculosis
    drug resistance, 14
    infection, 41
    preventing, 15
    resistance to heat or
        chemicals, 100
    special testing, 42
Mycoplasma pneumoniae
    infection, 45
N95 personal respirator, 29,
    43, 93, 95
National
    Clinicians' Postexposure
        Prophylaxis Hotline, 64
    Institute for Occupational
        Safety and Health, 90,
        93, 98, 141, 144, 148,
        149, 161
    Institute of Allergy and
        Infectious Diseases,
        161
necropsy room worker
    and *Mycobacterium*
        tuberculosis, 42
necrotizing fasciitis, 50
needle
    blunt-tip, 129
    butterfly-type, 131
    disposable, 131

hypodermic, 131
protective shield, 129
retractable, 129
needleless intravenous
system, 129
needlestick
and hepatitis B virus, 58
and hepatitis C virus, 61
and human
immunodeficiency
virus, 64
and *Mycobacterium
tuberculosis*, 41
immediate first aid, 78
injury log, 149
negative-pressure room and
chickenpox and
disseminated zoster, 72
measles, 71
rubeola, 30
tuberculosis, 43
Neisseria meningitidis
(meningococcus)
infection, 16, 45
postexposure prophylaxis,
46
transmission, 24, 29
NIOSH. *See* National
Institute for Occupational
Safety and Health
noncritical-class device, 30,
119, 121
nonlipid virus, 99
norovirus infection, 68
nosocomial
infection, endogenous, 22
pneumonia, preventing,
16
obesity, high-risk host, 25
Occupational Safety and
Health Administration, 26
regional offices, 162
requirements
biohazard warning
label, 135
bloodborne pathogen
exposure, 79, 80

employee medical
records, 148
engineering controls,
128
Exposure Control Plan,
141
eye protection, 92
gloves, 89
handwashing, 82
hazard communication,
137, 143
housekeeping, 120
injury logs, 147
masks, 92
personal protective
equipment, 86, 88
protective clothing, 97
regulated waste, 133
resuscitation devices,
94
sharps, 129
training, employee, 144
workplace inspection,
138
work-practice controls,
128
ocular herpes, 63
Office Sterilization and
Asepsis Procedures, 161
organ transplant and
cytomegalovirus, 57
infection, 25
Toxoplasma gondii, 51
oropharyngeal anthrax, 34
OSHA. *See* Occupational
Safety and Health
Administration
other potentially infectious
materials, definition, 29
otitis media, and
*Streptococcus
pneumoniae* infection, 49
oxacillin. *See*
Staphylococcus aureus
drug resistance
packaging instruments, 109
parachlorometaxylenol, 87

parenteral exposure, 77
parotitis, and mumps, 67
paroxysm, and pertussis, 35
pathogen
drug resistance, 14
infectivity, virulence, and
toxicity, 25
resident, 21
transient, 21
patient
history, 26
transport, 30, 71, 72
penicillin resistance, 14
peracetic acid, 103, 105
percutaneous exposure, 63,
77
personal protective
equipment, OSHA
requirements, 86, 88
personal respirator, 28, 34,
43, 95
N95/HEPA, 93
pertussis, 35
pharyngitis, 50
phenolic, 119
phlebotomy site, 25
pneumococcal infection. *See*
*Streptococcus
pneumoniae*
(pneumococcus)
pneumonia and
adenovirus infection, 55
Chlamydia pneumoniae
infection, 36
hospitalization, 16
Legionella pneumophila
infection, 41
measles, 71
Mycoplasma pneumoniae
infection, 45
respiratory syncytial virus
infection, 69
Staphylococcus aureus
infection, 48
*Streptococcus
pneumoniae* infection,
49
pocket mask, 94

poliovirus
  infection, 16
  poliomyelitis, 68
  resistance to heat or
    chemicals, 100
postexposure prophylaxis
  Baccilus anthracis, 34
  Bordetella pertussis, 35
  Clostridium botulinum, 37
  Corynebacterium
    diphtheriae, 38
  hepatitis A virus, 57
  hepatitis B virus, 60
  human immunodeficiency
    virus, 64
  Neisseria meningitidis, 46
  OSHA requirements, 79,
    80
  rubeola virus, 71
  variola virus, 74
precautions. See Standard;
  Airborne; Contact; Droplet
pregnancy and
  cytomegalovirus infection,
    56
  hepatitis E virus infection,
    62
  influenza virus infection,
    66
  rubella virus infection, 70
  rubeola virus infection, 71
  Toxoplasma gondii
    infection, 51
  varicella zoster virus
    infection, 72
presoaking instruments, 106
prion, 99, 103
prosthesis, dental, 125
protective
  clothing, 96
  coverings, 121
  gloves, 86
pulmonary disease, high-risk
  host, 25
pumice, 126
purpura, 39
radiation treatment, 26
radiograph film, 136

rag wheel, 101, 125
record keeping
  employee medical
    records, 147, 148
  employee training
    records, 149
  injury logs, 147
  regulated waste
    disposals, 147
  sterilization monitoring,
    147
red bag, 134
regulated waste
  containers, 134
  disposal, 135
  liquid, 136
  OSHA definition, 133
  OSHA requirements, 133
renal disease, high-risk host,
  25
reporting. See case reporting
reservoir. See cycle of
  infection
resident pathogen, 21, 22
respirator. See personal
  respirator
respiratory
  syncytial virus infection,
    69
  therapy equipment, 118
respiratory tract secretions
  containing
    adenovirus, 55
    Bordetella pertussis, 35
    Chlamydia pneumoniae,
      36
    Corynebacterium
      diphtheriae, 38
    cytomegalovirus, 56
    influenza viruses, 66
    mumps virus, 67
    Mycobacterium
      tuberculosis, 23, 41
    Mycoplasma pneumoniae,
      45
    Neisseria meningitidis, 45
    poliovirus, 68

respiratory syncytial virus,
    69
rubella virus, 70
rubeola virus, 71
Streptococcus
    pneumoniae, 49
Streptococcus pyogenes,
    50
varicella zoster virus, 72
variola virus, 73
resuscitation device, OSHA
    requirements, 94
rheumatic fever, 50
rhinitis, 91
rhinovirus, resistance to heat
    or chemicals, 100
risky sex, 25
rubber
  dam, 96
  stopper and alcohol, 119
rubella virus infection, 70
  preventing, 16
rubeola virus. See also
    measles (rubeola)
  infection, 71
  prophylaxis, 71
safe zone, 130
salad bar contamination, 24
saliva containing
    cytomegalovirus, 56
    herpes simplex virus, 63
    mumps virus, 67
    Neisseria meningitidis, 45
Salmonella, 29
  in food, 24
  infection, 46
  resistance to heat or
    chemicals, 100
salmonellosis, 46
scalpel, 101, 130
scarlet fever, 50
scoop technique, 132
self-infection, 81
semen containing
    cytomegalovirus, 56
    hepatitis B virus, 58
    human immunodeficiency
      virus, 63

semicritical-class instrument or device, 100, 101, 102, 104, 123
sepsis syndrome, 26
sharpening stone, 131
sharps
    and bloodborne pathogen exposure, 77
    as regulated waste, 133
    avoiding injury, 128
    injury log, 148
    safety devices, 129
Shigella sonnei
    in food, 24
    infection, 47
shigellosis, 47
shingles. See herpes zoster
shorting electrical switches, 120
sickle cell anemia, high-risk host, 25
sink trap, 136
skin infection, and Staphylococcus aureus, 48
skin lesion/rash, 91, 143
smallpox, 73
smoking restriction, 98
soap dispenser, 84
sodium hypochlorite, 118, 119, 125, 126
soil containing Toxoplasma gondii, 51
sonographic vaginal probe, 118
source patient, 58, 80
speculum, 101
splint disinfection, 119
spontaneous abortion and rubella virus infection, 70
    rubeola virus infection, 71
sporicidal, 87, 118
spray-wipe-spray method, 120
sputum, 42, 44
Standard Precautions, description, 27
Staphylococcus aureus

drug resistance, 14, 29, 30, 48, 87
infection, 48
resident nasal, 22
resistance to heat or chemicals, 100
steam sterilization, 103, 106
sterilants, 100, 102
sterile
    gloves, 90, 113, 124
    handpiece head cover, 114
    sharpening stone, 131
    tissue, 21, 22
    towel, 85, 113
    water, 113, 124
sterilization
    and instrument lubrication, 106
    cycle, 110
    failure, 110
    monitoring
        biological, 111
        chemical, 112
        physical, 113
    precleaning
        checklist, 107
        ultrasonic cleaner, 107
    presoaking and corrosion, 107
    steps, 106
steroids, and Staphylococcus aureus infection, 48
stethoscope disinfection, 119
stillbirth, and rubella virus infection, 70
stone cast, 125
storing sterilized instruments, 113
strep throat, 50
Streptococcus pneumoniae (pneumococcus)
    drug resistance, 14
    infection, 16, 49
    vaccine, 49

Streptococcus pyogenes (group A streptococcus) infection, 50
suctioning, 77, 92
surface disinfection, 120
surgical
    cap/hood, 97
    gloves, 89, 90
    hand scrub
        iodophor, 87
    incision, 25
    mask, 29, 30, 43, 45, 92, 93, 95
    site infection, preventing, 15
surgical hand scrub, 84, 85
susceptible host, 22, 25
suturing, 77, 130
sweat, 28
swivel arm, 122
synovial fluid containing hepatitis B virus, 58
Taiwan acute respiratory agent, 36
tears, 25
teeth, extracted, 103, 128
telephone contamination, 24
thermometer disinfection, 119
thrombotic thrombocytopenic purpura., 39
toxic shock-like syndrome, 50
Toxoplasma gondii
    infection, 51
    toxoplasmosis and toxoplasmic encephalitis, 51
training, employee
    methods, 145
    OSHA-required, 142, 144
    records, 149
transient pathogen, 21
transmission modes, 22
Transmission-Based Precautions, 28
transplant surgery, 26
transport. See patient

contaminated instruments and devices, 117
contaminated laundry, 97
regulated waste, 133, 135
triclosan, 87
tube head, 122
tuberculosis, 41
    infection control checklist, 43
    isolation room requirements, 43
    multidrug-resistant, 44
    precautions against, 28
ultrasonic
    cleaner, 107, 108
    scaler tip, 101
ultraviolet lamp, 43
Universal Precautions, 27, 97, 135
unsaturated chemical vapor, 103, 106
urine containing
    cytomegalovirus, 56
    poliovirus, 68
utility gloves, 90
vaccination, 27
    checklist, 163, 164, 165, 166, 167, 168
    childhood, 15
    health care worker, 15
vaccine
    adenovirus, 56
    anthrax, 34, 163
    bacille Calmette Guérin, 44, 168
    diphtheria, tetanus, and pertussis, 163
    Haemophilus influenzae type B, 164
    hepatitis A, 164
    hepatitis B, 59, 164
    hepatitis B declination statement, 59
    influenza virus, 16, 67, 165
    measles, mumps, and rubella, trivalent, 71

measles, mumps, and rubella, trivalent, 166
meningococcus, 16, 167
mumps virus, 68
pneumococcus, 16, 49, 167
poliovirus, 16, 69, 168
rubella virus, 16, 70
rubeola virus, 71
smallpox, 168
tetanus-diphtheria, 38, 168
varicella zoster virus, 16, 73, 163
vaginal secretion containing
    herpes simplex virus, 63
    human immunodeficiency virus, 63
vancomycin. See enterococci drug resistance
varicella zoster virus
    infection, 29, 72
    preventing, 16
    postexposure prophylaxis, 73
variola virus infection, 73
vector-borne transmission, 25
ventilation, 17
    and sterilant use, 102
    and tuberculosis, 43
    devices, 88, 94
vesicle fluid containing
    herpes simplex virus, 63
    varicella zoster virus, 72
vinyl gloves, 90, 91
vomitus, 27
waste. See regulated waste
water
    -based lubricant, 106, 108, 114
    containing
        Cryptococcus neoformans, 24
        Cryptosporidium parvum, 39

Legionella pneumophila, 41
stains on new gloves, 88
sterile, definition, 113
wax bite/rim, 125
West Nile virus, 25
wheezing, 91, 92
whooping cough, 35
work restrictions
    adenovirus infection, 56
    cryptosporidiosis, 39
    diphtheria, 38
    Escherichia coli infection, 40
    giardiasis, 40
    hepatitis A, 57
    hepatitis B, 58
    herpes simplex virus infection, 63
    human immunodeficiency virus infection, 64
    influenza virus infection, 67
    meningococcal meningitis, 46
    mumps, 67
    pertussis, 35
    respiratory syncytial virus infection, 70
    rubella virus infection, 70
    rubeola virus infection, 71
    salmonellosis, 47
    Staphylococcus aureus infection, 48
    Streptococus pyogenes, 50
    tuberculosis, 44
    vaccinia vaccine recipient, 74
    varicella zoster virus infection, 72
work-practice controls, 128
x-ray head disinfection, 119

Reference List for Further Study

1. Bolyard EA, Tablan OC, Williams WW, et al. Guideline for infection control in healthcare personnel, 1998. *Infection Control and Hospital Epidemiology.* June 1998;19(6):407-463; <u>and</u> *American Journal of Infection Control.* June 1998;26(3):289-354. See also: www.cdc.gov
2. Garner JS, CDC, Hospital Infection Control Practices Advisory Committee. Guideline for isolation precautions in hospitals. *American Journal of Infection Control.* February 1996;24(1):24-51. See also: www.cdc.gov
3. CDC. Guidelines for preventing the transmission of *Mycobacterium tuberculosis* in health-care facilities, 2005. *Morbidity and Mortality Weekly Report.* December 30, 2005;54(RR-17):1-141.
4. Mangram AJ, Horan TC, Pearson ML, et al. Guidelines for the prevention of surgical site infection, 1999. *Infection Control and Hospital Epidemiology.* April 1999;20(4):247-278, and *American Journal of Infection Control.* April 1999;27(2). See also: www.cdc.gov
5. CDC. Guidelines for prevention of intravascular catheter-related infections. *Morbidity and Mortality Weekly Report* August 9, 2002;51(RR-10):1-26.
6. CDC. Recommendations for preventing transmission of infections among chronic hemodialysis patients. *Morbidity and Mortality Weekly Report.* April 27, 2001;50(RR-05):1-43.
7. CDC. Guideline for hand hygiene in health-care settings. *Morbidity and Mortality Weekly Report.* October 25, 2002;51(RR-16):1-44.
8. CDC. Management of multidrug-resistant organisms in healthcare settings, 2006. www.cdc.gov
9. CDC. Guidelines for infection control in dental health-care settings—2003. *Morbidity and Mortality Weekly Report.* December 19, 2003;52(RR-17):1-61.
10. CDC. Updated U.S. Public Health Service guidelines for the management of occupational exposures to HIV and recommendations for postexposure prophylaxis. *Morbidity and Mortality Weekly Report.* September 30, 2005;54(RR-09):1-17.

11. CDC. Immunization of health-care workers: recommendations of the Advisory Committee on Immunization Practices and the HICPAC. *Morbidity and Mortality Weekly Report.* December 26, 1997;46(RR-18):1-41.

12. MMWR quick guide: recommended immunization schedules for persons aged 0-8 years–United States, 2007. *Morbidity and Mortality Weekly Report.* January 5, 2007;55(MM-51&52):Q1-Q4..

13. CDC. Public Health Service Task Force recommendations for the use of antiretroviral drugs in pregnant HIV-infected women for maternal health and interventions to reduce perinatal HIV-1 transmission in the United States. *Morbidity and Mortality Weekly Report.* January 30, 1998;47(RR-02):1-30. See update: January 24, 2001 at www.hivatis.org

14. CDC. Prevention of pneumococcal disease: recommendations of the Advisory Committee on Immunization Practices. *Morbidity and Mortality Weekly Report.* April 4, 1997;46(RR-08):1-24.

15. CDC. Preventing pneumococcal disease among infants and young children: recommendations of the Advisory Committee on Immunization Practices. *Morbidity and Mortality Weekly Report.* 2000;49(RR-09):1-38.

16. CDC. Guidelines for prevention of nosocomial pneumonia. *Morbidity and Mortality Weekly Report.* January 3, 1997;46(RR-01):1-79.

17. CDC. Prevention and control of influenza: recommendations of the Advisory Committee on Immunization Practices. *Morbidity and Mortality Weekly Report.* July 28, 2006;55(RR-10):1-42.

18. CDC. Prevention and control of meningococcal disease, and meningococcal disease and college students: recommendations of the Advisory Committee on Immunization Practices. *Morbidity and Mortality Weekly Report.* June 30, 2000;49(RR-07):1-20.

19. CDC. Poliomyelitis prevention in the United States: updated recommendations of the Advisory Committee on Immunization Practices. *Morbidity and Mortality Weekly Report.* May 19, 2000;49(RR-05):1-22.

20. CDC. Control and prevention of rubella: evaluation and management of suspected outbreaks, rubella in pregnant women, and surveillance for congenital rubella syndrome. *Morbidity and Mortality Weekly Report.* July 13, 2001;50(RR-12):1-23.

21. CDC. Prevention of varicella: updated recommendations of the Advisory Committee on Immunization Practices. *Morbidity and Mortality Weekly Report.* May 28, 1999;48(RR-06):1-5.

22. CDC. Guidelines for environmental infection control in health-care facilities. *Morbidity and Mortality Weekly Report.* June 6, 2003;52(RR-10):1-42.

23. Department of Labor, OSHA. 29 CFR Part 1910.1030. Occupational exposure to bloodborne pathogens; final rule. *Federal Register.* December 6, 1991;56(235):64175-64182.

24. Chin J., editor. *Control of Communicable Diseases Manual.* 17th edition. Washington, DC: American Public Health Association. 2000.

25. U.S. Army Medical Research Institute of Infectious Diseases. *Medical Management of Biological Casualties Handbook.* 4th edition. February 2001. MD: Frederick (Fort Detrick): USAMRIID. www.usamriid.army.mil/education/bluebook.html

26. Young LS, Rubin RH. Introduction. Chapter 1 in: Rubin RH, Young LS, editors. *Clinical Approach to Infection in the Compromised Host.* 3rd edition. New York, NY: Plenum Medical Books; 1994.

27. Larson EL. APIC guideline for handwashing and hand antisepsis in health care settings. *American Journal of Infection Control.* August 1995;23(4):251-269.

28. Weinstein RA. Infection control in the hospital. Chapter 98 (pp.586-589) in: Isselbacher KJ, Braunwald E, Wilson JD, et al, editors. *Harrison's Principles of Internal Medicine,* 13th edition. New York, NY: McGraw-Hill; 1994.

29. Berkow R, editor-in-chief. *The Merck Manual of Diagnosis and Therapy.* 16th edition. Rahway, NJ: Merck & Co; 1992:5, 13-20.

30. Pearson ML, CDC. Guideline for prevention of intravascular device-related infections. *American Journal of Infection Control.* August 1996;24(4):262-293.

31. Thomas CGA. *Medical Microbiology.* 6th edition. London, England: Baillière Tindall; 1988:14, 63-64.

32. CDC. Transmission of HIV possibly associated with exposure of mucous membrane to contaminated blood. *Morbidity and Mortality Weekly Report.* July 11, 1997;46(27):620-623.

33. CDC. Weekly update: West Nile virus activity–United States, October 31-November 6, 2001. *Morbidity and Mortality Weekly Report.* November 9, 2001;50(44):983.

34. Brachman PS. Epidemiology of nosocomial infections. Chapter 1 in: Bennett JV, Brachman PS, editors. *Hospital Infections.* 3rd edition. Boston, MA: Little Brown and Company. 1992.

35. Sands KE, Bates DW, Lanken PN, et al. Epidemiology of sepsis syndrome in eight academic medical centers. *Journal of the American Medical Association.* July 16, 1997;278(3):234-240.

36. Stone R. Search for sepsis drugs goes on despite past failures. *Science.* April 15, 1994;264(5157):365-367.

37. CDC. Notice to readers: interim guidelines for investigation and response to *Bacillus anthracis* exposures. *Morbidity and Mortality Weekly Report.* November 9, 2001;50(44):987-990.

38. CDC. *Epidemiology and Prevention of Vaccine-Preventable Diseases.* "The Pink Book." 6th edition. Washington, DC: Public Health Foundation. January 2000.

39. Fraser RS, Colman N, Müller NL, Paré PD. *Diagnosis of Diseases of the Chest.* 4th edition. Philadelphia, PA: WB Saunders. 1999.

40. Sunenshine, RH, McDonald, LC. Clostridium difficile-associated disease: new challenges from an established pathogen. *Cleveland Clinic Journal of Medicine.* February 2006;73(2).

41. Juranek DD. Cryptosporidiosis: sources of infection and guidelines for prevention. *Clinical Infectious Diseases.* August 1995;21(Supplement 1):S57-61.

42. Nash TE, Weller PF. Protozoal intestinal infections giardiasis, cryptosporidiosis, trichomoniasis, and others. Chapter 179 (p.911) in: Isselbacher KJ, Braunwald E, Wilson JD, et al, editors. *Harrison's Principles of Internal Medicine.* 13th edition. New York, NY: McGraw-Hill; 1994.

43. CDC. *Core Curriculum on Tuberculosis: What the clinician should know.* 4th edition. 2000.

44. Beers MH, Berkow R, editors. *The Merck Manual of Diagnosis and Therapy.* 17th edition. Whitehouse Station, NJ: Merck Research Laboratories. 1999.

45. Kramer F, Sasse SA, Simms JC, et al. Primary cutaneous tuberculosis after a needlestick injury from a patient with AIDS and undiagnosed tuberculosis. *Annals of Internal Medicine.* October 1, 1993;119(7/part 1):594-595.

46. Collins CH, Grange JM. Tuberculosis acquired in laboratories and necropsy rooms. *Communicable Disease and Public Health.* September 1999;2(3):161-167.

47. Fujiwara PI. *Clinical Policies and Protocols.* 3rd edition. Bureau of Tuberculosis Control, New York City Department of Health. June 1999.

48. CDC. *TB facts for health Care Workers.* January 2000. www.cdc.gov

49. CDC. Treatment of tuberculosis. *Morbidity and Mortality Weekly Report.* June 20, 2003;52(RR-11):1-77.

50. Leake JAD, Perkins BA. Meningococcal disease: challenges in prevention and management. *Infections in Medicine.* 2000;17(5):364-377.

51. Facts and Comparisons. *Drug Facts and Comparisons.* 54th edition. MO: St. Louis. 2000.

52. Sherertz RJ, Bassetti S, Bassetti-Wyss B. "Cloud" health-care workers. *Emerging Infectious Diseases.* March–April 2001;7(2).

53. Fiore AE, Levine OS, Elliott JA, et al. Effectiveness of pneumococcal vaccine for preshool-age children with chronic disease. *Emerging Infectious Diseases.* November-December 1999;5(6). Centers for Disease Control and Prevention.

54. Fein A, Grossman R, Ost D, et al. *Diagnosis and Management of Pneumonia and Other Respiratory Infections.* OK, Caddo: Professional Communication, Inc. 1999. www.pcibooks.com

55. Bartlett JG, Dowell SF, Mandell LA, et al. Practice guidelines for the management of community-acquired pneumonia in adults. *Clinical Infectious Diseases.* August 2000;31:347-382.

56. CDC. Nosocomial group A streptococcal infections associated with asymptomatic health-care workers—Maryland and California. 1997. *Morbidity and Mortality Weekly Report.* March 5, 1999;48(8):163-164.

57. Bisno AL, Gerber MA, Gwaltney JM, et al. Diagnosis and management of group A streptococcal pharyngitis: a practice guideline. *Clinical Infectious Diseases.* September 1997;25(3):574-583.

58. Kasper LH. *Toxoplasma* infection and toxoplasmosis. Chapter 177 (p.904) in: Isselbacher KJ, Braunwald E, Wilson JD, et al, editors. *Harrison's Principles of Internal Medicine,* 13th edition. New York, NY: McGraw-Hill; 1994.

59. CDC. Preventing congenital toxoplasmosis. *Morbidity and Mortality Weekly Report.* March 31, 2000;49(RR-02):57-75.

60. CDC. *Adenoviruses.* June 1999. www.cdc.gov/ncidod/dvrd/nrevss/eadfeat.htm

61. Department of Defense. *U.S. Department of Defense Contracts."* No. 461-01. September 26, 2001. www.defenselink.mil/news

62. CDC. Two fatal cases of adenovirus-related illness in previously healthy young adults—Illinois, 2000. *Morbidity and Mortality Weekly Report.* July 6, 2001;50(26):553-555.

63. CDC. Civilian outbreak of adenovirus acute respiratory disease, South Dakota, 1997. *Morbidity and Mortality Weekly Report.* July 17, 1998;47(27):567-570.

64. CDC. Prevention of hepatitis A through active or passive immunization: recommendations of the Advisory Committee on Immunization Practices. *Morbidity and Mortality Weekly Report.* October 1, 1999;48(RR-12):1-37.

65. Hadler SC, Francis DP, Maynard JE, et al. Long-term immunogenicity and efficacy of hepatitis B vaccine in homosexual men. *New England Journal of Medicine.* 1986;315(4):209-214.

66. CDC. Recommendations for preventing transmission of human immunodeficiency virus and hepatitis B virus to patients during exposure-prone invasive procedures. *Morbidity and Mortality Weekly Report.* July 12, 1991;40(RR-8):1-9.

67. CDC. Recommendations for prevention and control of hepatitis C virus (HCV) infection and HCV-related chronic disease. *Morbidity and Mortality Weekly Report.* October 16, 1998;47(RR-19):1-39.

68. CDC. *Viral Hepatitis C Fact Sheet.* August 25, 2001. www.cdc.gov/ncidod/diseases/hepatitis/c/fact

69. Terrault NA, Wright TL. Viral hepatitis A through G. Volume 2, Chapter 68 in: Feldman M, Scharschmidt BF, Sleisenger MH, editors. *Sleisenger and Fordtran's Gastrointestinal and Liver Disease: Pathophysiology, diagnosis, management.* 6th edition. Philadelphia, PA: WB Saunders; 1998.

70. CDC. *Hepatitis G Fact Sheet.* 1998.

71. Robbins DL. Human herpesviruses: research, and threats to health professionals. *General Dentistry.* October 1994;42(5):418-422.

72. Fauci AS, Lane HC. Human immunodeficiency virus (HIV) disease: AIDS and related disorders. Chapter 279 (p.1571) in: Isselbacher KJ, Braunwald E, Wilson JD, et al, editors. *Harrison's Principles of Internal Medicine,* 13th edition. New York, NY: McGraw-Hill; 1994.

73. Hodes DS. Respiratory infections and sinusitis. Chapter 25 in: Katy SL, Gershon AA, Hotez PJ. *Krugman's Infectious Diseases of Children.* 10th edition. St. Louis, MO: Mosby-Year Book, Inc. 1998.

74. CDC. Measles, mumps, and rubella—vaccine use and strategies for elimination of measles, rubella, and congenital rubella syndrome and control of mumps: recommendations of the Advisory Committee on Immunization Practices (ACIP). *Morbidity and Mortality Weekly Report.* May 22, 1998;47(RR-8):1-57.

75. CDC. Norovirus in Healthcare Facilities Fact Sheet. December 21, 2006. www.cdc.gov

76. Katy SL, et al. Rubella (German measles). Chapter 26 in: Katy SL, Gershon AA, Hotez PJ. *Infectious Diseases of Children.* 10th edition. St. Louis, MO: Mosby-Year Book, Inc. 1998.

77. Katy SL, et al. Measles (rubeola). Chapter 16 in: Katy SL, Gershon AA, Hotez PJ. *Infectious Diseases of Children.* 10th edition. St. Louis, MO: Mosby-Year Book, Inc. 1998.

78. Kinchington PR. Latency of varicella zoster virus: a persistently perplexing state. *Frontiers in BioScience.* February 15, 1999;4:d200-211.

79. Department of Labor. OSHA. 29 CFR Part 1910. Personal protective equipment for general industry; final rule. *Federal Register.* April 6, 1994;59(66):16334-16364.

80. Donowitz LG. *Infection Control for the Health Care Worker.* 2nd edition. Baltimore, MD: Williams and Wilkins. 1995.

81. Cohen BI, Pagnillo MK, Musikant BL, et al. Evaluation of the electrical permeability of hand creams applied to latex gloves. *General Dentistry.* November-December 1997;592-598.

82. Food and Drug Administration and Health Industry Manufacturers Association. *Gloves: Information about medical gloves.* 1992.

83. National Institute for Occupational Safety and Health. *NIOSH Alert: Preventing allergic reactions to natural rubber latex in the workplace.* DHHS Publication. 97-135. June 1997.

84. Schwimmer A, Massoumi M, Barr CE. Efficacy of double gloving to prevent inner glove perforation during outpatient oral surgical procedures. *Journal of the American Dental Association.* February 1994;125:196-198.

85. Patton LL, Campbell TL, Evers SP. *General Dentistry.* January-February 1995:22-26.

86. Safadi GS, Safadi RJ, Terezhalmy GT, et al. Latex hypersensitivity: its prevalence among dental professionals. *Journal of the American Dental Association.* January 1996:127:83-88.

87. Molinari JA. Practical infection control for the 1990s: applying science to government regulations. *Journal of the American Dental Association.* September 1994;125:1189-1197.

88. CDC. *NIOSH-Recommended Guidelines for Personal Respiratory Protection of Workers in Health-care Facilities Potentially Exposed to Tuberculosis.* 1992.

89. Chen SK, Vesley D, Brosseau LM, et al. Evaluation of single-use masks and respirators for protection of health care workers against mycobacterial aerosols. *American Journal of Infection Control.* April 1994;22(2):65-74.

90. Department of Labor, OSHA. Occupational exposure to tuberculosis. 29 CFR Part 1910. *Federal Register.* October 17, 1997;62(201):54260-54263.

91. Willeke K, Qian Y. Tuberculosis control through respirator wear: performance of NIOSH-regulated respirators. *American Journal of Infection Control.* April 1998;26(2):139-142.

92. ADA Roadmap to CDC Guidelines for Infection Control in Dental Health-Care www.ada.org/prof/resources/topics/cdc/index.asp#roadmap.

93. Gutmann ME. Air polishing: a comprehensive review of the literature. *Journal of Dental Hygiene.* Summer 1998;72(3):47-56.

94. Granzow JW, Smith JW, Nichols RL, et al. Evaluation of the protective value of hospital gowns against blood strike-through and methicillin-resistant *Staphylococcus aureus* penetration. *American Journal of Infection Control.* April 1998;26(2):85-93.

95. Miller CH, Palenik CJ. *Infection Control and Management of Hazardous Materials for the Dental Team.* St. Louis, Mo: Mosby-Year Book, Inc; 1994.

96. Rutala WA. APIC guideline for selection and use of disinfectants. *American Journal of Infection Control.* August 1996;24(4):313-342.

97. Favero MS, Bond WW. Chemical disinfection of medical and surgical materials. In: Block SS, editor. *Disinfection, Sterilization and Preservation.* 4th edition. Philadelphia, PA: Lea & Febiger; 1991:621.

98. Velji AM, Hoeprich PD. Sterilization and disinfection. Chapter 19 in: Hoeprich PD, Jordan MC, Ronald AR, editors. *Infectious Diseases.* 5th edition. Philadelphia, PA: JB Lippincott Company. 1994.

99. Spaulding EH. Chemical disinfection of medical and surgical materials. In: Lawrence CA, Block SS, editors. *Disinfection, Sterilization, Preservation.* Philadelphia, PA: Lea & Febiger. 1968:517-531.

100. CDC. Recommended infection-control practices for dentistry, 1993. *Morbidity and Mortality Weekly Report.* May 28, 1993;42(RR-8):1-11.

101. Lado EA, Stout FW. Sterilizer monitoring: option or responsibility? *General Dentistry*. November-December 1994;42(6):560-563.

102. Dept. of Veterans Affairs, ADA, and Dept. of Health and Human Services. *Infection Control in the Dental Environment*. 1992.

103. Rhame RS. The inanimate environment. Chapter 15 (p,321) in: Bennett JV, Brachman PS, editors. *Hospital Infections*. 3rd edition. Boston, MA: Little Brown and Company. 1992.

104. Goodman HS, Carpenter RD, Cox MR. Sterilization of dental instruments and devices: an update. *American Journal of Infection Control*. April 1994;22(2):90-94.

105. Jacobs PT. *Sterrad*TM *Sterilization System: A new technology for instrument sterilization*. Advanced Sterilization Products. 1994.

106. Crow S. Peracetic acid sterilization: a timely development for a busy healthcare industry. *Infection Control and Hospital Epidemiology*. February 1992;13(2):111-113.

107. Miller CH. Cleaning, sterilization and disinfection: basics of microbial killing for infection control. *Journal of the American Dental Association*. January 1993;124:48-56.

108. Martin MA, Wenzel RP. Sterilization, disinfection, and disposal of infectious waste. Vol. 2, Chapter 280 in: Mandell GL, Bennett JE, Dolin R, editors. *Mandell, Douglas, and Bennett's Principles and Practice of Infectious Diseases*. 4th edition. New York, NY: Churchill Livingstone. 1995.

109. Food and Drug Administration, Center for Devices and Radiological Health. Sterilants and High-Level Disinfectants Cleared by FDA in a 510(k) as of 10/28/97 with General Claims for Processing Reusable Medical and Dental Devices. http://www.fda.gov/cdrh/ode/ germlab.html

110. Martin MA, Reichelderfer M. APIC guideline for infection prevention and control in flexible endoscopy. *American Journal of Infection Control*. February 1994;22(1):19-38.

111. Roberts C, Antonoplos P. Inactivation of HIV type 1, hepatitis A virus, respiratory syncytial virus, vaccinia virus, herpes simplex virus type 1, and poliovirus type 2 by hydrogen peroxide gas plasma sterilization. *American Journal of Infection Control*. April 1998;26(2):94-101.

112. Steris Corporation. Steris System 1TM. Technical Data Monograph. 1988.

113. Vassal S, Favennec L, Ballet JJ, et al. Hydrogen peroxide gas plasma sterilization is effective against *Cryptosporidium parvum* oocysts. *American Journal of Infection Control*. April 1998;26(2):136-138.

114. Rutala WA. New disinfection and sterilization methods. *Emerging Infectious Diseases*. March-April 2001;7(2).

115. Bradley CR, Babb JR, Ayliffe GAJ. Evaluation of the Steris System 1 peracetic acid endoscope processor. *Journal of Hospital Infection*. 1995;19:143-151.

116. Miller CH. Sterilization: disciplined microbial control. In: Runnells RR, guest editor. *The Dental Clinics of North America: Infection Control and Office Safety*. Philadelphia, PA: WB Saunders Co; April 1991;35(2):339-355.

117. Cottone JA, Terezhalmy GT, Molinari JA. *Practical Infection Control in Dentistry*. Malvern, PA: Lea & Febiger; 1991.

118. Burkhart NW, Crawford J. Critical steps in instrument cleaning: removing debris after sonication. *Journal of the American Dental Association*. April 1997;128:456-463.

119. Association for the Advancement of Medical Instrumentation. *Steam Sterilization and Sterility Assurance in Office-Based, Ambulatory-Care, Medical and Dental Facilities*. Arlington, VA: AAMI; 1993.

120. Kolstad RA. The emergence of load-oriented sterilization. *Journal of the American Dental Association*. January 1994;125:51-54.

121. Bryce EA, Roberts FJ, Clements B. When the biological indicator is positive: investigating autoclave failures. *Infection Control and Hospital Epidemiology*. September 1997;18(9):654-656.

122. Association of Operating Room Nurses. Event-related sterility. *AORN Journal*. June 1994;59(6):1313-1314.

123. Schwartz R, Davis R. Safe storage times for sterile dental packs. *Oral Surgery, Oral Medicine, Oral Pathology*. 1990;70(3):297-300.

124. Muscarella LF. Letters to the editor. *American Journal of Infection Control*. April 1998;26(2):153-156.

125. Department of Labor. Needlesticks and Other Sharps Injuries; Final Rule," *Federal Register*. January 18, 2001;66(12):5318-5325.

126. National Institute for Occupational Safety and Health, CDC. *Alert. Preventing Needlestick Injuries in Health Care Settings*. DHHS (NIOSH) Publication 2000-108. November 1999. www.cdc.gov/niosh

127. Nicol GH. *Florida's New Biomedical Waste Law: A practice guide for dentists*. 1997. Tallahassee, FL: Florida Dental Association.

128. CDC. Public Health Dispatch: Potential risk for lead exposure in dental offices. *Morbidity and Mortality Weekly Report*. October 12, 2001;50(40);873-874.

129. ADA Council on Scientific Affairs. Dental mercury hygiene recommendations. *Journal of the American Dental Association*. July 1999;130:1125-1126.

130. Department of Labor, OSHA. 29 CFR 1910. et al. Hazard communication; final rule. *Federal Register*. February 9, 1994;59(27):6126-6184.

131. OSHA. *Inspecting for Job Safety and Health Hazards*. OSHA Fact Sheet 93-02. January 1, 1993.

132. Runnells RR, Powell GL. Managing infection control, hazards communication, and infectious waste disposal. In: Runnells RR, guest editor. *The Dental Clinics of North America: Infection Control and Office Safety*. Philadelphia, PA: WB Saunders Co; April 1991;35(2):299-308.